The TRUTH about CANCER
Apollo Pampallis

The TRUTH about CANCER & its PREVENTION

Apollo Pampallis
and 6 Nobel Laureates

Copyright

Copyright © by Apollo Pampallis 2015
The TRUTH about CANCER & its PREVENTION
2nd Edition 2016

First published in South Africa – September 2015
The right of Apollo Pampallis to be identified as the author of the work has been asserted in accordance with the Copyright Act 98 of 1978.

All rights reserved, whether the whole or part of the material is concerned. ©

Contact:
Apollo Pampallis
+27 71 322 0582
booksthatheal@gmail.com

DTP:
Clive Thompson
International Professional Book Designer
https://www.getclive.com
email: cliveleet@mweb.co.za
cell: 083 761 0698 studio: 031 207 4884

Cover Photo:
Clive Thompson

Dedication

I dedicate this book to the loving memory of my father Peter, dearly beloved by all who were touched by his loving smile and unconditional love and kindness, who succumbed to cancer barely six months after being diagnosed. Tragically, customs confiscated a remedy I had imported, without informing me. By the time I realized what had happened, it was too late for my father. Due to my insufficient knowledge then, I could not help him. The same remedy subsequently gave my father's friend three years of quality living after five doctors gave him a maximum of three weeks to live.

My pact with my dying father was to ensure that I do whatever I could to prevent any other person from going through what he did, by awareness and consciously preventing cancer as well as the artscience of its transcendance.

And that is precisely what I have striven to do. As a significant part of my Life Purpose, I have dedicated myself to helping people prevent cancer and guiding them to heal themselves, casting off cancer once diagnosed, through writing, workshops, and consultations, whether in person or internationally through Skype.

Αιώνια σου η μνήμη, Μπαπ.

Disclaimer

*Legal disclaimer: Author has no prescriptive authority and recommendations reflect author's opinion. Some products may require prescription where you reside. No products are 'prescribed' or claimed to heal anything. Other products to those referred to by the author sold by the same vendor are not necessarily endorsed by the author. All purchases are the decision and responsibility of the purchaser.
E & OE

"Do not let either the medical authorities or the politicians mislead you. Find out what the facts are, and make your own decisions about how to live a happy life and how to work for a better world."

Linus Pauling, *Ph.D., World's greatest contemporary Medical Researcher, Philanthropist and two-time Nobel Prize winner*

Thank You

I have indeed been blessed with exceptional people in my life who made this book possible.

Chloë

I would like to thank my daughter Chloe for always believing in and encouraging me, even in times where I have not succeeded to pull through for her. and I am moved in anticipation of the blessing you will bestow upon humanity in your own special, unique and unprecedented way . Never ceasing to fascinate me, Chloe dreamt up this and other images of the Sacred Delphic Epsilon, the green growing tip her personal touch, being named after the Greek goddess of our Great Earth Mother.

Photini Economou

For your tireless efforts in promoting an awareness that cancer CAN be prevented and treated after losing her brother to cancer. Her facebook group, "The Truth about Cancer, Prevention is Better than Cure is jambpacked with useful, mostly free information essential for our times.

Mom

Mom, thanks for your support in rough times, your reading of the book and helpful suggestions.

Clive Thompson

If you want any DTP work, anywhere in the world, without a doubt, this is the man to turn to if you want talent, dedication and integrity.
www.getclive.com

Contents

Part One –
Setting the Stage   **17**
1. Cancer and You   17
2. Questions Demanding Answers   21
3. Our Objective   25
4. What is Cancer   26
5. The Business of Cancer   32

Part Two –
Causes and Prevention of Cancer and   **37**
Introducing Two Causes and their
Resolution in Eight Areas of Your Life.
1. Food   38
2. Oxygen, Acidity and Sugar   64
3. Emotions   72
4. Electromagnetism   90
5. Hormones   97
6. The Physical Body   110
7. Acidity and Fungus   124
8. Medicines and Antibiotics   129

Part Three –
Closing Our Case   **149**
1. A Cure to Die For   150
2. The "War Against Cancer"   155
3. The Heart of the Matter   159
4. Zooming Out   162

Part Four –
References and Resources   171

Maximizing Your Benefit

A great deal of research and thought has gone into this book. It had to be truly holistic, fully scientific and totally verifiable, yet reader friendly. On the one hand, I wanted to put in as much information as I could, but on the other, I realised that few people would commit to reading a huge book. So I trimmed it as much as possible, to a readable and affordable size for most people, but with the access to resources of a book ten times its size.

Despite this, you may find some repetition which is unavoidable and indeed desirable, as all aspects of this book are inextricably linked, proving and reinforcing one another in creating a Whole. I have also found that repeating "unorthodox" concepts from different perspectives increases the likelyhood of them been considered, understood and thus accepted.

Claims in this book are referenced by superscripts. All references and recommended resources at the time of writing are instantly and freely accessible via links in the resources list or hyperlinks in the electronic version, and the book's web page, instead of hiding behind difficult, expensive, or impossible-to-obtain books and journals. You needn't check out all the references. I have listed multiple references in most instances from various sources, for two reasons: Firstly, to show that the point made is not just the perspective of just one person or organisation, and secondly, many links may fail over time, as webmasters change their sites, and sites disappear. There is also the ominous threat to future access to information on the net. Wherever possible I have provided free video links where you can actually experience the doctor, or other authority, speak. Remember, all truth is realised, not told, imposed or believed. Personal freedom and empowerment means that *you* are responsible for realising your own truth.

All recommended resources that are not free, are people and companies that I have found to be of integrity, offer exceptional goods or services and the best value for money. The links to such resources from the website will change with time, according to my ongoing research, saving you the time, risk and expense of doing your own research.

Of course, I do not control outside links and cannot be held responsible should they at some time fail. Nor can I guarantee that you will experience the same excellent service that I had with vendors. However, I am open to feedback and shall endeavour to continuously update for the best resources at any time.

I would recommend that you first read the book so that you retain focus and continuity, returning to check out the resources.

You will also be entitled to register for the book's community, which means that you will be continuously updated with the latest findings, be able to interact with other readers, and receive relevant news as well as preferential treatment and rates for various goods and services.

Keep this book accessible to reinforce and motivate you and share, lend and give it away generously, knowing that by so doing you will sooner or later be preventing much suffering, saving lives and sparing families from tragic losses and financial ruin.

The electronic version may not be "locked" or "copy protected", so that you can download it onto any devices that you may have, but please do not pirate it, as funds from this book are dedicated to the upliftment of humanity, and your support is integral to the fulfilment of this purpose.

For companies and organizations that care for their employees as well as philanthropic organizations, bulk orders can be made.

If you are a health practitioner, product or service-provider in agreement with the philosophy of this book, approach me to list your services on the book's website and discuss ways of networking. We must work together to serve humankind.

Be open to, but do not blindly believe any word, written or spoken, from whatever source (including this book), without subjecting it to inner scrutiny. All beliefs are mere opinions determined by time and space perspectives and not always validated by personal experience, but to the contrary, beliefs determine and mould your experience. Take (back) your personal responsibility to verify and select the beliefs which serve you best.

Truth is neither told nor believed, it is *realized*. Thus beliefs and blind faith are the biggest enemies of (self) realization. As the Delphic Oracle taught: "Know[ing] Thyself" is the Truth, as the external world is merely a projection or reflection of our feelings, fears, aspirations and beliefs.

© Apollo J Pampallis. Permission to use passages from this book granted subject to reasonable conditions upon written request to booksthatheal@gmail.com.

Prologue

Welcome! Before we continue, let me repeat the following: None of what some may consider controversial views here are originally or exclusively mine, but of others who are academically, legally and experientially qualified to make them, for the most part the highest authorities in their fields, mostly within the medical establishment. Where views expressed are due to my own belief, opinion, or experience, these are explicitly identified as such. I encourage you to validate any claim with the given references, freely accessible on the internet at the time of writing and by all means do your own research. I am not a doctor and have no prescriptive authority, legal responsibility or right over your health. The conclusions must always be yours. Don't ever let anybody, including me, deprive you of this right and responsibility.

There are many good books written about cancer prevention, each touting a particular approach. However, this book is, I am told, the most truly holistic guide to cancer prevention. It begins with the true hidden causes of cancer, exposes fraudulent claims, explains the dynamics of disease in a scientific but reader-friendly way and applies this new insight with practical steps to optimal health in all areas of your life.

"The greatest mistake in the treatment of diseases is that there are physicians for the body and physicians for the soul, although the two cannot be separated." – **Plato**.

Instead of Plato's insight being recognized and acted on over the millennia, physicians now increasingly dis-integrate the body-mind complex and specialize in ever-smaller parts of the body, as if the body (and mind) does not operate as an integral whole. This is why a medical treatment for one "part" invariably poisons another, so that the "treatment" for asthma could harm the heart, medication for which could lead to kidney issues and so on, resulting in "cures" creating conditions progressively worse than the original "problem". Likewise, in psychiatry drugs for depression, or alleged "ADD", which drug manufacturers candidly admit in their package inserts may lead to depression, "sudden death" violence and suicides!

To this I would add another grave mistake which we have taken for granted and that is emphasis on the physician to "know", from a theoretical point of view, (i.e. 'theorize') what is happening to a patient. This is in contrast to the approach of a true healer who has always been one who guides you to *experientially understand* what is happening to, or through you, (their patient), thus empowering you, not to "get rid" of the disease, nor to restore yourself to a state before you experienced (physically manifested) the sickness, but to understand *how and why* you hosted the condition in the first place and so empower you to choose healthier alternatives for healthier outcomes. Both health and disease are personal issues and response-abilities too important to delegate to anyone else, regardless of their title, or to the extent they are learned in the ever-changing "scientific facts" and belief systems of the time.

Thus diseases such as cancer give us a choice: to fear and resist to our mortal peril, or to understand, transcend and attain a state of health far greater than that which brings or brought about the condition in the first place. In other words, we don't try to kill the messenger, but take heed of, and act upon the message (pain, discomfort) so that it is no longer relevant or necessary – preferably before the disease becomes (physically) manifest, let alone life threatening.

I facilitate this best through my body-mind therapies which I have done for people from all five continents, an experience too profound to be described in words, and which I am often called upon to do after speaking and workshop tours. What happens cannot be limited or reduced to a "technique" such as aromatherapy, shiatsu, Swedish massage or various other "energy healing" modalities (all of which I have taught before they became formalized in South Africa), but a Unique Healing

Experience at every encounter which cannot simply be taught, let alone "franchised", but learnt only after many years of disciplined dedication. Having said that, I *do* teach the arts of Therapeutic Massage for therapists and healers, as well as Intimate Massage, a *must* for any couple to optimize their relationship in every way.

In response to requests by medical and non-medical health practitioners, I am in the process of creating higher order integrative methodologies which promise to greatly enhance whatever modalities they are using in their practices. Details of these will be made available upon request and in our newsletter. Body-mind therapies constitute an essential part of my Transcendent Protocol for everyone, including those going through the cancer experience. Doctors generally attempt to treat the disease a person has. Following Hippocrates' dictum, I treat and empower the person the disease has, (and we *all* experience dis-ease to various extents, be it emotional, spiritual and/or physical) through personal consultations (in person or on Skype), talks and workshops.

Every attempt is made in this book to at least question dangerous beliefs that most of us take for granted, but no attempt is made to replace them with another "belief system". To the contrary, it is my conviction that the greatest gift that anyone, but especially a healer can bestow, is the gift of empowerment by exposing disinformation and faciliting the freedom to choose, so that you may connect with your own Inner Truth, which ultimately provides the best cure for every ill in the world, including cancer. In fact, freedom to choose (and humour) are faculties which distinguish us from animals or automatons. Herein lies true healing, as beautifully expressed in the Ancient Greek word and transcendent concept of freedom, *"eleutheria"* (ελευθερία), a compound word meaning the unimpeded channeling (έλευση/ eleusi) of divine (θείου/theio) loving, fulfilling, reconciling energy ('Ερως/Eros). However, this can only be achieved once we are liberated from the slavery of imposed, but consciously and unconsciously accepted, blinding and enslaving beliefs, many of which we dogmatically cling to, at a terrible cost to our happiness and even our very lives.

16 The TRUTH about CANCER

Part One

Setting the Stage

1. Cancer and You　　　　　　　　　17
2. Questions Demanding Answers　　21
3. Our Objective　　　　　　　　　　25
4. What is Cancer　　　　　　　　　26
5. The Business of Cancer　　　　　32

1. CANCER AND YOU

This book may be the wisest and most cost-effective investment you have ever made and quite possibly life-saving for you and anybody in your care, as you shall soon discover. *Congratulations!*

Cancer is everybody's concern, with the probability of you dying of cancer rapidly rising from the current "one in three" chance, to "one in two" chance in the next few years. There are many studies showing increased incidences, particularly in women, that have caused various agencies to make similar frightening predictions. According to the International Agency for Research on Cancer (IARC), a branch of the World Health

Organization (WHO), "Global cancer rates are expected to increase 50% by the year 2020."[1] Other reports from different sources predict a 70% increase in the next 20 years.[2]

There is even documented evidence backing an outrageous claim that there is a plan to exterminate 80% of the world's population. If articles such as this one[3] (of many obtainable via Google) convince you, or if you are aware of the "Georgia Monument" (USA) prescribing an ideal world population of half a billion, let it further strengthen your resolve to be one of the 20%.

Moreover, even without a genocide plan, we must remember that in order for any ecosystem to exist, whenever any species grows out of control and threatens environmental sustainability and survival, something will happen to control it. In the case of humans now, the "ecosystem" is the whole world. Never before has so much environmental damage been done and so extensively, so that for the first time in recorded history the whole planet's life-support system is endangered. But remember as always, it's survival of the fittest – "the fittest", in this case, being those who are aware of what is happening and who act appropriately and in such a way as to not be one of the 80% "lemmings". In reading this book, you are knocking on the door of the "20% Club". By putting it into practice, you qualify for full membership.

Before we proceed: For those of you who fearfully embrace the belief that cancer runs in your family DNA, both celebrated cancer therapist Dr Leonard Coldwell and Prof. Bruce Lipton, the world's most ground-breaking cell biologist (having worked with cloning and stem cells in the 1970s, decades before his colleagues had even heard of them), have shown that this belief is mistaken. Dr Coldwell, who broke the "genetic predisposition to cancer" fallacy on both sides of his family, saving his mother from a liver cancer death sentence, and obliterating the disease entirely from his family, is living proof of this, as he states in this five minute video.[4]

Prof Lipton's "new" science of epigenetics (επί/epi=above, beyond genetics) at Stanford University has consistently and conclusively proved that although genes may "predispose", they do not "determine". Like being given a loaded gun, *you decide* whether to lay it down, hide it, defend yourself, murder somebody or commit suicide with it.

Watch the free videos by Prof Lipton[5] and Dr Coldwell. You may well want to order their respective books.[4B, 5B]

Lipton's findings concur with those of the outspoken Dr. Samuel Epstein, Cancer Prevention Coalition founder and Professor Emeritus at the University of Illinois, who concluded that less than 2% of cancers have a hereditary component.[6] These findings *perfectly* complement those of chiropractor, Dr Austin Sanford, DC, B.S., current President of Healthcare Intervention Inc., who stated: "We are waiting on a miracle drug when 98% of cancers are caused by lifestyle choices and can be avoided altogether."[7]

When a top biologist, a top medical doctor and a top chiropractor all break the mould of their professions, the mould of a paradigm and of "common sense" to arrive at precisely the same conclusion *(to 1% concurrence!)*, – that it is we who decide whether to succumb to, in fact to *create* cancer or not – dare we dispute it?

There can be only one question: What are these life choices? Join me in identifying the "wrong, bad and cancerous" life choices that our leaders, our education, our communities and even our own parents have taught us and which we have been passively accepting as "the obvious way to live", so that we can then be in a position to replace them with informed, wise and life supporting beliefs, thoughts and commitments.

In 1971, when cancer was nowhere near as rampant as it is now, President Nixon pledged to "rid the world of this scourge", pouring millions of taxpayer's dollars into corporate pharmaceutical companies for alleged "cancer research". Since then, four things have happened:

1. The incidence and death from cancer, particularly lung cancer, has risen and is sharply rising, *despite* a dramatic

decrease in smoking.

2. The money committed to this research has gone solely to "Big Pharma" and the world's largest chemical cartels like the Nazi affiliated IG Farben / Hoechst / Bayer syndicate and their progeny, notably "Agent Orange" Monsanto, world leaders in GMOs (genetically "modified" organisms), and others in this field. (Hereafter I use the term "genetically mutated" to more objectively describe the insidious "pirating" of biologically legitimate forms with genes from entirely different life forms, something which, unlike hybridisation, could never occur naturally).

3. Not only has genuine (non-Big Pharma) research been denied support, but no expense of our tax money has been spared to relentlessly persecute, even "eliminate", pioneers in new effective paradigms of cancer treatment, both within and outside the medical profession; and in ridiculing, outlawing, and squashing many effective cancer treatments/cures "legally" through government agencies such as the FDA (which "coincidentally" has the same leadership as Monsanto at time of writing) and the DEA in the U.S., as well as other policy-making and professional organizations and governments worldwide, controlled directly or indirectly by the drug (pharma) cartels.[8]

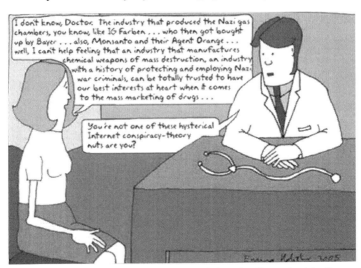

(cartoon from: http://www.whale.to/b/nazi_allopathy.html)

4. Despite all alleged research, claims and promises, pharmaceutical medicine is no closer to a cancer cure, having succeeded only in prolonging patients' suffering, always at great financial expense. Healthy people don't buy many drugs, but dead people buy nothing. And desperate, suffering people consume the most. Sales are optimized by maintaining a population healthy enough to generate money, but sick and brainwashed enough to depend on drugs and pay to keep their loved ones "alive" as long as possible, irrespective of the suffering they go through.

2. QUESTIONS DEMANDING ANSWERS

1. Are companies that pioneered chemical warfare, and that still poison people, animals, and the environment, ethically qualified to heal people from disease?
2. Why has the incidence of cancer (and many other diseases) risen so sharply *after* the declared "War on Cancer"?
3. Why is it that proven (and unproven, due to lack of research funds) non-pharmaceutical methods of treating cancer have been so relentlessly squashed by corporate controlled government agencies?
4. Why are medical personnel legally sponsored to dispense drugs with possible effects (euphemistically and slyly referred to as "side-effects") often worse than the condition treated, and which are very often themselves carcinogenic? Why do medical doctors withhold such information, and why do pharmacies often remove the information insert that accompanies drugs before handing them over, instead of making receipt of drugs conditional to the recipient user of legal age or guardian having read, understood and signed acknowledgement at the time of prescription and dispensing?
5. Why is there an offensive against vitamins, herbal remedies, and natural food and remedies under the *Codex Alimentarius*, a food and supplement trade restricting protocol which the UN is enforcing on the world, initiated by a (WWII) convicted war criminal, Fritz Ter Meer, ex-President of IG Farben? And why were officials in the same

company, who were found guilty of war crimes, released from jail and reinstated?

6. Why are alcohol and tobacco promoted when they are both highly addictive and dangerous, whilst the most therapeutic herb Cannabis (which is by nature not addictive as is alcohol, tobacco, caffeine, refined sugar, junk food, etc.) remains illegal?

Cannabis has now been proven not to be a "gateway drug" (to other substances) and it is one of the strongest known cancer preventatives and treatments, as well as found by many to be the safest and most effective treatment for ADD, glaucoma, and many other diseases when used responsibly. Yet it is banned, criminalised or (often ruthlessly) controlled, purely due to its euphoria-inducing effects which, incidentally, have none of the harmful and dangerous consequences of all the substances in parentheses in the previous paragraph. As such, nobody, and no organization, has a justifiable or ethical right to prohibit its use. In fact it's serotonin and melatonin-raising properties, without the "side-effects" (including suicide) of pharmaceutical Selective Serotonin Reuptake Inhibitors (or SSRI's), such as Prozac® and Zoloft®, make it a highly effective and far safer and less addictive alternative for psychiatric use where the latter are prescribed.[9] Notwithstanding this, I do not endorse its ingestion by smoking, as whilst not nearly as harmful or as carcinogenic as cigarette smoking, inhaling any smoke is unhealthy and potentially carcinogenic. Neither do I consider it to be a "cure-all", as with any herb its abuse or misuse can have deleterious effects, but there again this does not justify repressive legislation.There is nothing, including life-giving water and oxygen which is not toxix in excess

However, there is an even better substance for temporarily addressing depression, (no substance 'cures' depression-only therapeutic body-mind self-discovery does, in my experience); a highly recommended legal herbal supplement far outperforming pharmaceutical anti depressants and even Cannabis and the everpopular St John's Wort, with no undesirable "side" effects whatsoever, and with anti-carcinogenic effects to boot. It is the

South African plant *Sceletium tortuosum*, commonly known as "kanna," is used extensively by the indigenous Khoi and San people long before the arrival of the white man and the migration of the black man from the north nearly half a millennium ago. It can be further investigated and ordered here.[10]

It is we, the people of the world, who have allowed ourselves to be hypnotically conditioned to be naively trusting and gullible, unquestionably obeying our governments, schools, religions and the medical and other "authorities", even if the results are horrifically tragic to ourselves, our families, our communities, our countries, and the whole world. We have abdicated our personal response-ability, discernment, free will, integrity and faith in our own ability to reason, to politicians and multinational "elites" whose interests are blatantly in opposition to our planetary, national and personal well-being. This applies particularly to our acceptance of cancer as a "dread", "incurable" disease and subjugation to the most torturous and dehumanizing "treatments" for it. Official medical statistics themselves prove these treatments to be not only ineffective, but much worse than no treatment, as we shall see. Not only that, but we pay with all we have and even put ourselves into irrevocable debt for the dubious privilege of receiving such "treatments".[11]

There is no better definition for insanity, especially when "spontaneous remission," also referred to as "natural regression" (i.e., cancer recovery without treatment), occurs in at least 14%, up to 24%, even 27% (according to Dr Coldwell)[12] of patients, and recovery after chemo "therapy" occurs in only about 2%! So, with absolutely *no treatment* whatsoever, your chances of recovery are, according to official medical statistics, at the very least 12 percentage points better!

Statistics "proving" improved cancer recovery rates are misleading, as indirectly conceded in the U.S. government's official health website, which acknowledges that the cure rate has not increased since the 1950s. Modern allopathic treatment modalities may claim to have merely succeeded in protracting the patient's *miserable* survival, but you may find that "success rates" that were previously based on five-year survival rates have now been "revised" to three-year survival rates.[13]

According to the same government website, the "natural regression" rate of breast cancer is far greater than my 14% average stated above. It says: "The recent six-year Norwegian follow-up study on breast cancer in women also accepts the fact of *natural regression in one-fifth* (my italics) of the untreated cases that were followed up; the authors concluded that this may reflect the fact that these cancers are rarely allowed to follow their natural course." What a tragedy! So instead, with chemo, we now have a whole lot of amputee women and a survival rate of just over 2%! Note again that we are not talking about an "alternative" site, but the US National Library of Medicine page of the National Institutes of Health site.[14]

Many people try to justify "conventional medication" by relating the death of the late co-founder and head of Apple® Corporation, Steve Jobs, who purportedly refused medical treatment for pancreatic cancer and is alleged to have regretted it, only acceding to accepting it on his deathbed. However let's look at the facts: He lived for eight years with the cancer. How long do people diagnosed with pancreatic cancer survive on the prescribed chemo? Eight Years? Five years? Three years? Think again. Look up the American Cancer Association medical survival rates. You will be horrified.

In truth, Steve Jobs appears to have been receiving so called "alternative" therapies simultaneously with chemo, and my recent Google searches (mid 2014) had consistently yielded the top 5-6 sites attributing his death to chemo, radiation and surgery.[15] (However, due a radical shift in Google's search criteria this is no longer the case) The pancreas secretes insulin, thus regulating sweetness in the body. This sweetness has its psycho-spiritual counterpart as metaphorical "sweetness" in our lives. Perhaps before concluding this book, if you know anything about his life, you may also have a clue as to what may have been the cause of his cancer, and how it may have been addressed and transcended.

You, and nobody else, are responsible for your life. And nobody is as affected by, or cares about your health as much as you do. Act accordingly! My lobbing the ball of your health into your court may terrify you, but that is the only side in which you have control of it if you want to win. Here are some generic questions I have been asked with respect to cancer prevention in my face-to-face and Skype therapy and healing sessions.

1. What is cancer?
2. What successes have there been in the cancer industry?
3. What causes cancer?
4. What are the precursors of cancer?
5. How can we eliminate, minimize, and compensate for carcinogens?
6. What can I do if I "have" cancer?
7. What can I do, it runs in the family? (You already know the answer to that).

If I gave you the answers in point form you would not accept them from where you now stand. And if you did, it would be on blind faith. I don't want you to believe anything or anyone, including me, without reason. The answers to all the above questions will emerge in the pages to come.

The final decision, commitment, and responsibility for your health are, however, yours.

3. OUR OBJECTIVE

The objective of this book is to empower you with sufficient knowledge and insight, leading to the ability to make wise, responsible choices in terms of your own and your dependents' health.

No mere knowledge derived from any book, including this one, will prevent cancer. However, if you conscientiously *take consistent action* with the simple, practical, and very doable guidelines set forth, you will most certainly make yourself practically, if not fully, cancer proof, almost as a "side-effect" of dramatically improved emotional, spiritual, and physical health.

When you complete this book, you will also have an idea of which areas of your life you need to focus on, and give special attention to, as we are all unique. How our health degenerates into disease is not the same for all of us. That is why each one of us requires a different intervention and/or different approaches and emphases. This was known to Hippocrates 2,600 years ago when he said that ten people with the same sickness would receive ten different treatments, because "you don't treat the disease the person has, but the person the disease has".

In addition, you will find all the resources you need, and a whole lot more, on the website of this book, and directly accessed by links on electronic editions. All the resources, whether free or charged by an independent vendor, have been created or carefully selected to ensure that you get the best and latest information on the Internet at any point in time, saving you time, money, effort, and the risk of dealing with unknown parties. These resources represent over 30 years of ongoing research in proactive health, off and online, now accessible at a click of your mouse.

If you have a product or service relevant to the objectives of this book, please contact me. This outreach cannot be done alone. My purpose is to network and cross-refer with other like-minded people and also create a directory of practitioners to serve them and clients/patients alike.

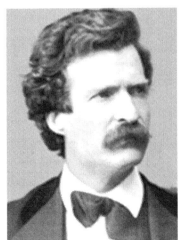

So to to our next chapter to address our first question

4. WHAT IS CANCER?

"It's not what you don't know that hurts you. It's what you 'know', but just ain't so"
— **Tom Sawyer**
(Mark Twain)

Four 'Wise' Blind Men encountered an elephant. The one, touching the trunk, fearfully screamed: "It is a serpent." The second, grasping its leg, felt great security and happily announced: "'Tis an ancient rough-barked tree," immediately evoking the feelings of stability and all the blessings that trees provide. The third, at the tail, sneered at the ignorance of the other two, as he amorously fantasized about the "lovely maiden whose flowing hair he clutched."

Most renditions of this story forget to mention the fourth man who, before even reaching the elephant, stumbled upon a pile of its manure, but had the good humour to laugh it off. "You guys are nuts. This whole elephant thing is a pile of shit."

(Adapted with gratitude and respect from the work of John Saxe whose original rendition was more elegant and whose emphasis slightly different, but by no means less important).

Which man had, not necessarily the truest, but the most functional or useful concept of an elephant, leading to the most appropriate action of calm retreat?

The man at the trunk raised his stick to strike out in an attempt to kill the "snake".

The one at the leg prepared to lie down to rest beneath his "tree".

The one at the tail was ready to follow it upward to kiss the "maiden's mouth".

...while the one that stumbled upon the dung simply walked away.

What would you, with the benefit of sight, have done?

Which man would have been most open to learning the truth?

Each one of the men emotionally anchored his belief with emotions of fear, the sense of security or passion respectively, except for the man who never even arrived at the elephant, who didn't even touch it. What be-LIE-fs have you invested in, solidified and identified with through partial/prejudiced information, fear, a (false) sense of security, and misplaced passion?

It is precisely those ideas, people, and institutions that will betray you.

Blindness is a condition of not being able, or *willing*, to see. Although blindness is related to eyesight, most sighted people are blinder than the blind. We are, to a great extent (far more than you can imagine), prisoners of our beLIEf systems, believing unquestionably what we have been told, despite often glaring evidence to the contrary. If I keep repeating myself on this, rest assured I cannot repeat it enough times, including to myself!

Is the Earth flat? Obviously. Ask any builder or farmer.
Is the Earth round? Obviously. Ask any sailor or pilot.
Is your mother-in-law a lovely person? "You must be joking!" I hear you say.
Is your mother a lovely person? "Of course!" says your dear spouse.

What we perceive as "truth" is almost, if not always, nothing other than a subjective belief, whether it be a "world view", "national view", "ideological viewpoint", religious dogma, "class perception", academic "fact", or your own individual synthesis of the above, none of which bear any relationship to an "objective reality". Conversely, your "truth" has more to do with yourself than the object of your perception (onto which you project your reality, i.e. "projection").

Let's look at the "official definitions" of cancer. According to the Oxford English Dictionary, cancer is:
1. A disease caused by an uncontrolled division of cells in a part of the body; a malignant growth or tumour resulting from such a division of cells.
2. Something evil or destructive that is hard to contain or eradicate."

Now in this case, we all know this is not only obvious, but established indisputable fact.
Or is it? Any Newtonian scientist will tell you that. Today's medicine is based on the Newtonian Science of the human machine: that you are a physical body, a machine that is subject to accidents and illness due to external factors, inherent faults, or bad luck. There is however a problem here – Newtonian physics as a model of ultimate reality has been surpassed for almost a

century, and Newton himself had in any case never claimed to explain, let alone heal, living beings!

However, ask any "primitive" person or any modern quantum physicist alike, for you to see the folly of such backward logic of the Oxford definition. Abnormally behaving cells *don't cause disease.*

Dis-ease is what causes the abnormal cells!

That is exactly why metastasis (μετα/meta-στάση/stase = after-stop, i.e. cancer cells "moving" to another part of the body) is so common *after* surgery to remove cancer-afflicted tissue. It is logically absurd for something which is no longer present to move.

It is very seldom due to a surgeon's incompetence, although both the anaesthetic and the physical and emotional trauma of surgery considerably weaken the person and further compromise the immune system.

It is due to the cancerous state "deciding" to manifest in the body. So if all you do is simply take out the part of the body where it manifests, it will most likely (unless you simultaneously address root causes) simply manifest itself in another.

It has been claimed that, on a physiological level, tumours tend to have "anti-metastatic chemicals" that actually discourage metastasis (which makes good survival sense for the tumour, as other tumours would compete for resources, thus further compromising the host on which they feed, at the expense of the original tumour) and these antimetastatic properties are paradoxically removed together with the tumour at surgery.

If cancer cells are removed, how can they "move" to another part of the body? A breast cancer case study in India in 2014 showed that women with surgical removal/amputation of one breast were slightly *more likely* to have the cancer metastasize to the remaining breast, or another part of the body, than women without surgery (removal by scalpel) or radiation (removal by burning), leading the doctor to advise against it.[16] A most significant revelation which has been swept under the carpet. No subsequent study has succeeded in refuting these findings.

Ladies, in particular, take note! In order to restore a person to health, you don't treat the disease. Never! You treat the *person!* After all, it is the person that is sick, not the infection, or the virus, or the cancer, which is doing very well thank you!

In the same way, if you knock your head and have a bump on it, do you get a hammer to flatten the bump? When you burn your hand, do you take a pain pill, or do you remove your hand from the fire?

Is the bump or burn the cause, or the result of your problem? And is it true that the bump on your head is the wall's "fault" and the burn the fire's fault, or is it possibly due to your own actions and relationship to the wall and fire which should be reassessed?

Thus the pain of the bump and burn, respectively (like the tumour), are *not* the problems, but the messengers, making you aware, warning and directing you to stop, or change the way of doing certain things, before you clobber yourself to death or incinerate yourself.

Hellooooo, pharmaceutico-medical complex; is there anybody in?

(Interestingly, there is an increasing number of people who believe that the tumour itself is the body's way of 'quaranteening' cancerous energy , citing evidence that 'dispersed' cancers are more 'agressive' than cancers 'focussed' in tumours.)

Of course, the second part of the Oxford definition of cancer only reinforces the lie with an irrational, superstitious association with fear and evil.

It will become increasingly obvious to you how this "inverted logic" actually promotes disease rather than prevents or cures it.

So what is it that makes a few "over-enthusiastic rogue cells" multiply uncontrollably, eventually culminating in our death? Why should a surplus of life energy itself paradoxically lead to our demise? In fact, Moritz, in his book (which you may want to read),[17] presents cancer itself as a survival mechanism.[17] de Martini also fleetingly alludes to this possibility towards the end of his book *The Value Factor*[18] where he fleetingly integrates wealth with health.

If we momentarily let go of our fear-fixated beLIEfs and took a moment to listen to Mother Earth, is it possible that this is the question, the clue and the answer She is trying to give to the human race, as "rogue life forms", like the cancer cells, no longer in harmony with, but a deadly threat to, our environment? This video reference and articles may help clarify the question.[19] If we, as a species, are cancers of the Earth, are cancers of the body also trying to tell us something? Are both not one and the same thing; a case of the "outer"/macrocosm reflecting the "inner"/microcosm, and then reflected back? This is a question to which we return in the final chapter.

How do we perceive ourselves, and consequently how do we project this self-perception in our relationships with one another and with Mother Earth Herself?

1. Are we machines, dependent on outside factors, like how we are driven, and environmental conditions, and limited by the way we were made, like a car? Then we are separate units reliant on (the expertise of) others, medical "mechanics" and "panel beaters" and directed to medico-pharmaceuticals to survive.
2. Are we biological organisms, part of an infinitely intricate natural environment? Then we need to honour that environment and our place in it, and likewise acknowledge natural therapies that work directly on the body, spine, energy meridians (acupuncture), and natural remedies, as obvious choices to heal our body, which is a natural living being, an integral part of nature, not just a chemical concoction needing more chemicals. In this case, we need to rely on our "Head" (intellectual) faculty.
3. Are we Spiritual Beings? Then we are all expressions of God/s, of Ultimate Being. Our health then depends on our conscious awareness at all times to BE healthy "cells" of Creation/the Universe that we wish to express physically

within us – Spiritual Beings having a physical experience. For this we need to be free of our egos and rely on our Heart.

Which of the above three is your point of reference? If you would really like to benefit fully (and truly "holistically") in your life and from this book, I invite you to be open to all three perspectives. Any mapmaker will tell you that in order to create a map correctly, you need at least two points of reference, but to even begin to understand the human condition, a three-dimensional approach is the barest minimum. And what better way is there than starting from a point of reference where all three perspectives are in perfect agreement?

All three above perspectives agree that cancer is a condition whereby strong biological forces appear to be misdirected to create an unchecked proliferation of cells which cease to identify with, and differentiate themselves from, their host, living off it, and draining its resources, without giving anything but toxic waste back in return, until the organism of which they were once an integral part can no longer support them and dies. From this all-inclusive position on physical symptoms and diagnosis, each of the above three models (in progressive order) have valid contributions to make to the determination of initial causes and subsequent courses of action, as seen in *Part 2*.

5. THE BUSINESS OF CANCER

Is the cancer industry successful? You bet it is. It's a multitrillion-dollar industry in league with (and directly connected to) the war and chemical-industrial complex, employing hundreds of thousands of people directly and millions indirectly. Nothing would be as disastrous for this business as a widely recognized cure. This is why any such potential "threats" must be eliminated at all costs, where human values and human lives are literally sacrificed on the altar of the god of profit. Yes, literally.

Just as the monetary system is a worldwide Ponzi/pyramid scheme, with the U.S. Federal Reserve and in turn all other "National Banks" being privately owned and enslaving the world in a vicious cycle of ever-increasing debt (where the poison (debt) is inherent in the "medicine" (money), as each additional banknote printed incurs increasing worldwide debt),[20] so, in a similar scheme, the pharmaceutical system maximizes profits by ensuring a sick population (as we shall see) which, in turn, thoughtlessly and addictively depends on it to survive.

And just as the "Prohibition" of alcohol in the 1920s was a scam that gave birth to the mafia and other notorious crime syndicates, the present "War on Drugs" merely entrenches the treacherous legal pharmaceutical and CIA-run illegal drug trade, whilst prohibiting "perception unblocking" and psychedelic (meaning "soul-revealing") -ψυχή/psych=soul δηλ/del-=revealing substances such as Cannabis and LSD respectively.

Of course, neither of these can be patented and monopolized by the "legal" pharma drug or illegal CIA-run drug cartels.[21]

"Coincidentally", these two substances tend to open people's minds to question our programmed beliefs and social rules and, if used responsibly, have psycho-physical therapeutic qualities bar none, including successful treatment of alcoholism and other drug addiction (with LSD) and the treatment of many diseases, most notably cancer (with Cannabis). Cannabis is to date the most successful cancer remedy *as part of a holistic protocol* as I have seen in cancer sufferers who I have coached to successfully facilitate their healing and shall show further in a possible forthcoming book on cancer treatment.

To be more accurate, we should perhaps talk about *transcending* conditions like cancer, rather than "curing" or "treating" them, as will become clear as we progress through this book. You may choose to consult me directly if you are presently afflicted, not for 'cures', but for coaching you back to health through self awareness, using 'natural remedies' not as a 'cure' in themselves, but as a means to support this end. There are none so joyous as those who have accepted cancer and transcended it through personal awareness.

The pharmaceutical industry churns out "pharmaca". In Ancient Greek (directly, or indirectly through Latin), the universal

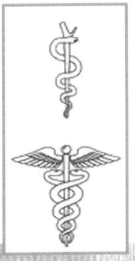

One Snake: *The Staff of Asclepius*
Two Snakes: *The Caduceus of Hermes*

language of science, φάρμακο/φαρμάκι (pharmaco/pharmaci) means "potion/poison", both Greek words differ only by one letter (as do the English), perfectly describing a "pharmaceutical" product, where a φαρμακεύς/pharmaceus is a poisoner, sorcerer.[22] (quite literally making a pharmaceutical company a

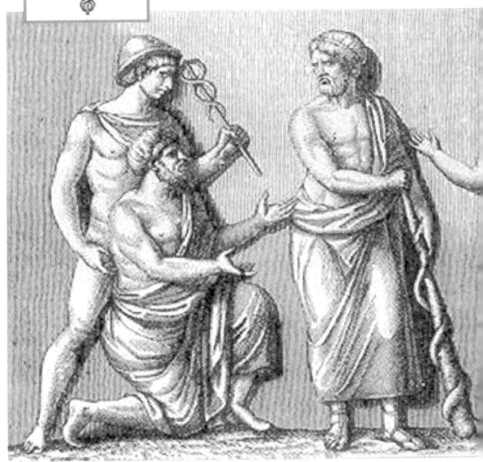

34 The TRUTH about CANCER

"wicked witches coven").

By contrast, a healing medicine is an "Iatriko" *(Ιατρικό, from "iasis/;ίασης=healing)*, dispensed by a "iatro" *(ιατρό)* – a health practitioner, as reflected in such modern words as paed*iatrist*/ic, pod*iatrist,* i*atrogenic* (sickness caused or 'birthed' by doctors), psych*iatrist/atric,* etc.

Furthermore, the symbol of the pharmaceutical industry appropriately is the winged caduceus with the two snakes of Hermes, god of (amongst other things) sorcerers, merchants and thieves. The symbol of Asclepius, god of healing by contrast, has a single snake ascending a natural, rough staff, symbolizing Life Energy (kundalini) ascending the spine. So can you see how modern day superstitious ignorance has us addicted to potions made by modern day sorcerer thieves in the misguided belief that we are taking an iatriko/ medicine? It doesn't get more literal or obvious than that!

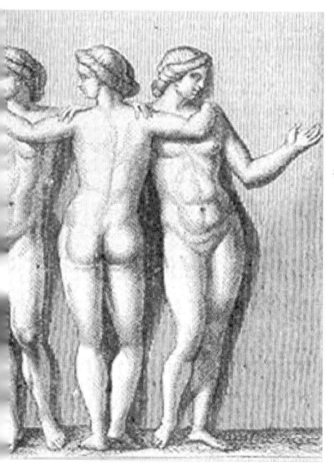

In the featured carved marble relief, we can see Hermes, with his twin-snaked caduceus on the left, facing Asclepius with his single-snaked staff. Note how Hermes and the crouching merchant pleaded with Asclepius from those times to commercialize healing arts and Asclepius's angry rejection. Asclepius rightly foresaw that the commercialization of the healing arts into a pharma/medical establishment would make Hermes (god of commerce,sorcerers and thieves) the god of the medical establishment, which totally contradicts the principle of empowering, helping, healing or at least doing no harm, as per the Hippocrateic Oath. By contrast, profit maximization involves creating and cornering a market, which means ensuring a constant supply of sick people and monopolistic access to the sick, through means now legally enforced due to bribing, blackmailing and control (euphemistically known as "lobbying") by the pharma multinationals of the governments of the world and relentless marketing "education" to doctors and victims alike.

Also significant are the three ladies with Asclepius. They are no common babes who would be taken in by Hermes's or the merchant's fancy chariot, pick-up lines or sales talk. They are the three Charities (Graces): Aglaia (Splendor), Euphrosyne (Mirth) and Thalia (Good Cheer), emphasizing that health is primarily not about absence of sickness, remedies, or even healthy eating, but first and foremost a way of living, a state of mind, living Life to the full with a joy that comes from within – something that, after thousands of years of the hijacking of human consciousness with poisonous thoughts and living, we are only beginning to re-member, and to real-ise, once again.

Before we look at the pharmaceutical industry and the medical treatment of cancer, could it be that the industry itself is a contributory cause, or even *the* major cause, of cancer? To answer this, we need to put everything into perspective, one step at a time, with new insights offered in Parts II and Parts III to follow.

Part Two

CAUSES AND PREVENTION OF CANCER
Introducing Two Causes In Eight Areas Of Your Life And Their Resolution

1. Food — 38
2. Oxygen, Acidity and Sugar — 64
3. Emotions — 72
4. Electromagnetism — 90
5. Hormones — 97
6. The Physical Body — 110
7. Acidity and Fungus — 124
8. Medicines and Antibiotics — 129

Cancer is a result of, firstly, poisons and secondly, imbalances (excess and deprivation), which we examine in eight interrelated areas of life, nearly all a result of modern living. Neutralize these and you eliminate the conditions for cancer. *Nothing can be simpler,* which is not to say that it's all easy in practice, but it's certainly simple in concept. You can be the judge of whether it is worth it.

Some people maintain that illness and cancer in particular, is the product of a toxic environment, including contaminated food, water, air and soil.

Others proclaim that illness and cancer are products of negative thinking and emotions: in other words, toxicity of the mind. In the old physics, one could say that one or both of the above are causative factors, but in quantum physics, we understand that just as the body-mind is one integrated whole, or unit, so too is the quality of our environment primarily the result of (the quality of) our thoughts and consequently actions. (And we in turn re-act to the environment we created in a vicious cycle). So although the outer is the reflection of the inner, we need to work on both simultaneously; not just re-act as victims, but respond positively (i.e. response-ably) to life circum-stances; to break the vicious cycle and create a virtuous cycle in its place, in time to save ourselves and our world.

1. FOOD

"Let food be your medicine and medicine be your food."
  – **Hippocrates, the Father of Medicine, 460-377 B.C.**

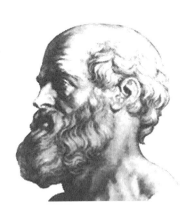

Food is what keeps us alive. If it is pure, wholesome, natural and good, it is the fuel of life, of optimal health, provided it is matched with an optimal state of mind.

However, "food" is no longer the pure gift of life, of Nature, upon which humanity has always thrived since its inception. The last hundred years or so has seen the quality of our food plummet, from a living gift of Mother Earth, to a deadly man-made concoction.

This is the inevitable result of a human race that has lost the plot, and lost the connection with Nature from which we have sprung and respect and love for our Primal Mother, Earth. Many reasons are given for this, including the Biblical reference that "man shall have dominion over the Earth", a tragic departure from all other religious and spiritual traditions that teach us to honour and respect Earth which unconditionally gives us life, home, nurturance and indeed our physical form. Indeed, that we belong to Earth and not vice versa.

Coupled with the "dominion" view is the prevailing Abrahamic religious tradition of oppressing the Female Principle in all its forms and its warring tradition based on notions of racial and/or ideological supremacy, condemnation and persecution of other peoples, nations and creeds as explicitly stated many times in the Talmud ("*goyim*"i.e "beasts"-), bible ("heathens") and Koran ("*kaffirs*/infidels").Besides being the 'spiritual creation' of divide and rule mentality and 'inventor' of racism, this starting point could only encourage a greedy, heartless patriarchal egocentricity whereby it is not only condoned, but even encouraged to rape and pillage fellow-man and the Great Earth Mother ruthlessly and endlessly in pursuit of personal economic profit with "divine sponsorship". Vast landscapes have been ravished for Her treasures and for monoculture, the planting of a single crop, year in, year out.

You cannot separate contempt of Mother Nature from contempt of her gifts, your own physical mother and ultimately from the contempt of self, which in turn is excplicity stated or at least implied in both ancient traditional wisdom and emerging sciences such as epigenetics as the primal direct and indirect cause of cancer.

Let us begin with processed "food". True food is a living input for a living being. Processed "food" is dead and full of chemicals that we should never eat. Most people don't even have a clue as to what they are eating in their "food", yet people we scorn as "primitive" are fully aware of exactly what they are eating, totally in tune with where it is from, the season and its place in Nature. Appreciative of the animal or even the plant they sacrificed or procured, and without being told to do so by religion, they make eating a sacrament. By contrast, all we know is in which aisle a package can be found in the supermarket, basing our selection on "brands" drummed into us, emphasized by bright artificial colourants, eye catching packaging, relentless hypnotic advertising, misleading assertions and blind, misguided faith.

Relatively few foods can be identified as directly carcinogenic. By far the majority are indirectly carcinogenic because they weaken and confuse the immune system and generally subvert a healthy biological system, optimizing conditions for fungal infestation preceding cancer-cell formation and proliferation. This happens mainly through creating hormonal imbalances and/or creating an acidic and anaerobic oxygen-starved cellular environment, as we shall see.

Dietary requirements are person-specific and not for generalization in books. So we focus here on overriding essential issues applicable to us all, such as alkalinity, balance and basic awareness of food toxicity – issues unknown or ignored by those of the 80% flock. Further to this, you are urged not to fall for "one-diet-suits-all" books and fads, but to turn to professional help if needed, as I encourage you to follow a diet optimal for you, within the context of the family or people with whom you live; guided, but not totally restricted, by the recommended diet for your blood type.

Parents happily treat their children to fizzy, carbonated sodas. The "fizz" is carbon dioxide, a poisonous waste product of living cells (not to mention many other toxic chemical ingredients out of which these often addictive drinks are made). When we breathe, the expulsion of CO_2 is even more immediately essential to our survival than the intake of oxygen! So why willingly drink the acid-creating toxin and poison the ones you love? This is particularly true of the most popular brown carbonated drink, with phosphoric acid and gm corn sugar or artificial sweeteners.[23]

Another pit of deceit into which many people willingly fall, is the "sugar-free" one, where synthetic "non-nutritive" sweeteners such as Aspartame® are used. Aspartame is the excrement of genetically mutated ("modified") bacteria. As such it is highly carcinogenic as well as ironically causing more obesity than sugar. Statistics show a huge rise in obesity *after* the introduction of synthetic "non-nutritive" sweeteners.[24] Sugar fattens, with refined sugar leading to a myriad of diseases from "AD(H)D to diabetes and even cancer due to its unnaturally high and unbalanced glycaemic index (quick release of energy/calories/kilojoules). Synthetic sweeteners are however far more poisonous and weight-gain therefrom is the least you should be concerned about with these highly carcinogenic sweeteners.[25]

It is recommended that sweetening of your food be done in moderation, with the healthiest sweeteners being raw honey, with its numerous health benefits, and the more compact and convenient zero-calorie *natural* sweetener, Stevia, best in liquid form (which does not have the additives and bitter aftertaste of Stevia powder), taken in drops, or even better, fresh or dried crushed leaves from your own stevia plant [26]

Remember, if we are going to be amongst the 20% of survivors of a "stealth" genocide, we need to have the courage, determination, perseverance and self-respect to do what the 20% does and not allow social pressure (need for approval), laziness or habit to passively do what the 80% do. I hope that by example you will influence others of the 80%, but always remember that whilst informing the wise may earn you gratitude, addressing fools will only earn you scorn. Indeed, as in most things, people most needing to learn are least likely to listen. Hence the saying attributed to Jesus: *"Cast not your pearls before swine."*

Bitter experience has taught me that trying to teach, heal and give everyone everything all the time ends up with me becoming exhausted and reaching practically no one, draining me of time and energy and unable to reach out to those who deserve the attention.

I had to learn the hard way, for when I was given advice to this effect, I rejected it, as I considered it arrogant. It is not. We all have gifts to offer the world, but a gift is only a gift to those who honour it and receive it as such. Otherwise such "gifts" are a wasted resource which could have been more constructively utilized where they would be honoured and put to good use.

Those interested in empowering themselves and their loved

ones and consider themselves worthy may take the initiative to read books such as this, attend (or organize) seminars in your area or arrange personal appointments including Skype sessions by contacting me by email or on http://cancerfree.cf

Life is a process of being open to learning through experience and through one another, something which we forget to our peril.

We are not the first "know it all", supposedly invincible culture. Many preceded us, and many will follow, the ego being what it is. The "invincible" Roman Empire died not as a direct result of Barbarian invasion, but by lead poisoning from its own "clever invention" of lead piping (*plumbus*, the Latin word for lead, is the root of the word "plumbing"). The elite were the first to succumb to lead poisoning, as they also fashioned their drinking vessels from high lead content clay, giving their skin a "shining" blue-silver sheen.[27] This is how the term "blue blooded" is linked to royalty (and not from "argyria", or excessive micro-silver ingestion from their cutlery, as believed by some).

But history, of course, keeps repeating itself (until we learn a lesson we shall tackle later in our book) and rather than project our own foolishness by judging the Romans, let's see where we are willingly poisoning ourselves. Amongst a myriad of poisons, let's look at our two favourite ones: Firstly, a poison even *more toxic* than lead and slightly less toxic than arsenic[28] (the second most deadly of all poisons), which people willingly consume under the false belief that it helps their teeth, the industrial pollutant and aluminium refining by-product, sodium or calcium fluoride, simply referred to as "fluoride".[29] Don't be fooled by "independent" studies, actually funded by pharmaceutical/ multinational/government interest groups.

This most successful of all rat poisons was originally used in Hitler's day to subdue a (human) population and its effect of calcifying (cirrhosis of) the pineal gland (a.k.a. the "master gland") in the centre of our brain, reducing people to mindless automatons, is well documented. There is no reason to suggest that it is not used for the same purpose right now,[30] as shown by academics such as Dr Bronner, a research chemist whose reputation is second only to that of Dr Yiamouyiannis PhD, the world's most prominent fluoride researcher and campaigner against its use, who died a suspiciously untimely death.

Furthermore, it does not help your teeth. To the contrary, it actually destroys teeth and bones and is linked to bone cancer as well as other forms of cancer,[31] as first proved by Dr Yiamouyiannis.[31e] Teeth with "fluorosis" are stained, ugly and very brittle. Many water filters do not remove fluoride, which is increasingly added to the water supply in the doubly deadly form of sodium fluoride, on the pretext that it is "good for you". Fluoride is cumulative. One tube of fluoridated toothpaste is more than enough to kill your toddler. Left mixed with some sweetening in a bowl, it is just as effective as any commercial fluoride rat poison.[32] Always use a fluoride-free toothpaste, which you most probably won't even find in your local supermarket, but in a health shop. Or make your own out of a combination of some, or all, of the following ingredients: bicarbonate of soda, diluted hydrogen peroxide (food grade only and very diluted as per instructions), and even charcoal. Experimenting with mixing and matching various toothpaste ingredients and the addition of various real herbal essences and flavours can be a fun, creative and a healthy family activity![33] Lastly, a natural way found to remove Fluoride from water[33d] and your body[33e]), using basil and turmeric respectively, the former a tasty, beneficial herb, the latter a mild spice and food colourant, as well as a potent anticarcinogen you should add to your food on a regular basis (at least the equivalent of a heaped teaspoonful a week; I sprinkle it and cinnamon lightly on my morning muesli, giving it added colour and aromatic taste).

A not so obvious poison trap is meat, which today is being eaten more frequently and in far greater quantities than at any other time in human history. To keep up with demand, minimize cost and maximize profit, animals are no longer being seen as living beings, but merely as inputs in food factories. The atrociously cruel conditions under which animals are raised and slaughtered, the toxic "feed" (as opposed to "real" food), hormones, antibiotics and other chemicals fed and injected into livestock (especially in the US, and Asia) would be unthinkable in any society with an inkling of sanity, humanity, ethics or compassion. The EU theoretically (but apparently not always in practice) bans (the Monsanto product) recombinant bovine growth hormone (rBGH), synthetic oestrogen, and other chemicals allowed in the U.S. Added to this, the adrenaline from the animal's continuously stressful and fearful life, particularly as it approaches slaughter, makes eating meat the way animals are now "manufactured" both ethically abominable and toxic to our health.[34] But it gets worse: we now even have genetically mutated ("modified"), teratogenic animals in the offing[35]

Although I am not a hunter and do not enjoy blood "sports", in all fairness, it is far more ethical and healthier to kill an animal suddenly, quickly and unexpectedly after it lived freely and naturally, unless it be raised humanely on small organic free-range farms.

Whilst not everyone is made out to be a vegetarian, we have never in history consumed meat in such quantities as we do today, and so we need to consciously moderate meat intake. Flesh-intense diets occur naturally only in environmentally challenged societies, where plants cannot grow, such as in Arctic Regions where only sea food and red meat are available.

If you do eat meat, ensure that it is from an organically raised animal, fed the vegetation it should be eating and not genetically "modified" soy and corn, or mince made from their sick and dead brethren (a common, if not standard commercial farming practice), or fishmeal. Choose "free range", not penned livestock, although even supposedly "free-range" animals are all too often packed so densely they can hardly move. Chickens have their beak tips cut off, an extremely cruel and painful procedure, so as not to be able to peck each other to death, an abnormal panic-induced behaviour brought about by overcrowding.[36]

Eating organic meat ensures that the animals are not raised on food unnatural to their species, genetically "modified" food, or any other non-organic feed and generally the animals are raised under more humane conditions. This is because organic farmers tend to be more compassionate and respectful of Nature

44 The TRUTH about CANCER

and cannot resort to drugs and antibiotics to prevent or "treat" sicknesses caused by overcrowding and stressful conditions. Such a farmer is Joe Salatin, who shows how to raise fowl and cattle in a biointegrated way simultaneously optimally and organically fertilizing his grazing land.[37]

Because organic farming does not trade off humane conditions or environmental concern for profit, organic foods cost more to produce, as later discussed, in the short term. But consider the relatively higher price you will pay for them as investments in your health as the real cost of eating non-organic food is far greater: in terms of your health, in environmental cost and in the medium to long term, in money.

We all have different dietary requirements based on many criteria including blood type, race, environmental factors, etc. Some people like to promote diets such a 100% raw vegetable and fruit diet, others a macrobiotic diet and proponents of such diets present living examples of people following their diets in radiant health.

The truth is that we are all different. While it is true that cooking destroys important enzymes in food, and for the most part decreases its nutritional and energy value, forcing any specific strict diet regimen may be right for some people, but not others, including you. For instance, although it may seem obvious to many of us that nutrition and enzyme-rich raw plant food is best, some people do not have the enzymes to digest it and must eat their food cooked. Another instance is that while nuts, being seeds, are generally amongst the most nutritious of all foods, packed with life energy, some of us are dangerously allergic to them.

In my opinion, a good starting point is a Mediterranean diet, which is tasty, balanced and nutritious, but with one caveat: minimize the amount of bread and in particular, minimize or eliminate wheat intake because of its high "heavy" gluten content.

There is a lot of confusion about gluten. Gluten is the "gluey" protein in all true grains which makes the dough stretchy and "plasticky". We have been eating bread and flour products for thousands of years without a problem. However, over the last century, wheat has been hybridized to contain much more, and much "heavier" gluten than in original wheat cultivars, which is helpful for baking, but too much for good health. As a result, a small but increasing number of people is now coeliac, which means that they have a dangerous, life threatening intolerance to all and any gluten, so that the tiniest trace of gluten can even kill them. Whilst not this bad, most of us are, to some extent, "gluten intolerant", with symptoms such as bloatedness, flatulence, listlessness, joint problems etc which may not be immediately attributed to it, considered "normal", or even passed unnoticed,[38] as we become increasingly out of touch with the vitality which is our birthright. Furthermore, gluten not only binds with and deprives us of essential proteins, but has been associated with stomach cancer, brain and neural problems and many other issues. Conversely, gluten avoidance has resulted in great improvements in epilepsy, autism and schizophrenia.

However, for most of us, whilst at least minimizing wheat flour bread is very important, total gluten avoidance is unnecessary, difficult, inconvenient and counterproductive, as processed food boasting to be "gluten free" may use chemical substitutes which are much more harmful to bind processed "food" in its place. These chemicals are often not even named, but simply referred to as "binding agents" or even "approved" binding agents.

As with "sugar free" foods, "vitamin fortified" processed breakfast cereals and other junk foods can be dangerously toxic.[39] "Fortifying" foods with vitamins removed/lost during processing does not "replace" lost vitamins which were originally in their natural, bioavailable form. Neither is the synthetic vitamin the same as that removed or killed in processing. For example, ascorbic acid is *not* the same as natural vitamin C, as is "fortified vitamin D" which is actually D2 and chemically different to natural vitamin D, and iron supplements which are toxic in excess.[39] According to this article,[39b] Nestle®even conceded that "vitamin fortification" is a marketing ploy to influence buying choices of mothers, not health motivated.

If you insist on eating wheat bread, ensure not only that it is made of whole-grain flour, which has the nutritious kernel or 'germ' and the essential roughage of the husk, and which is not chemically bleached/poisoned like white flour, but that it is stone ground. As for "brown" bread, more often than not it is white flour bread darkened with molasses, caramel (burnt sugar) or another colourant.[40] Acidic, sterile white flour stores better as it is less likely to be eaten by weevils and rodents, which are evidently smarter than us when it comes to nutrition.

Whole grain flour that is stone ground retains most of the seed's nutritive value, and even supplements it with minerals in minute particles of dolomitic calcium from the grinding stones. Nonetheless, even with stone ground wheat, the wheat germ oil is removed to extend the life of the flour, which is why it is good to add some drops of wheat germ oil obtainable at a health shop before use. Keep some refridgerated for up to a month, and freeze the rest.

Industrial flour mills, while much faster and more profitable to the merchants, operate at a high speed which literally "sterilizes" the flour, burning out the nutrients, leaving a "flour" which is literally dead, highly acidic and not fit for consumption. A rodent would rather eat the package than such flour. This assertion is further supported by a famous experiment where rats eating the box outlived all the rats eating the bran flakes contained therein.[41] As with the flakes, they'd probably only eat the flour if there is literally nothing else to eat. Reserve such flour for *papier mache*.

If you like bread, I would encourage you to make your own, and eat fresh, preservative free, mould-free bread made without chemicals, and out of grains other than wheat, such as rye, barley and spelt, all of which have a lower glial ("gluey") component in their gluten, which makes their gluten "lighter". Spelt is particularly low in gluten, and is considered gluten free by some as its gluten also has a very low glial content, making it acceptable for most gluten-intolerant people except coeliacs. It is also high in protein and alkalizing, due to plentiful magnesium, phosphorous, and calcium, essential elements sorely lacking in most of us. Indeed it is a wonder grain if eaten in moderation. [42]

If you have a bread-making machine, what can be more convenient than keeping a selection of low gluten bread premix packs in your freezer to pop into your bread machine at night for a fresh loaf the next morning? Store bread in brown paper packets, or even better, a drawstring cotton or linen bag, not plastic bags, especially when warm, as warm bread "sweats", and plastic traps the moisture, encouraging mould (fungus). (Supermarket bread comes in plastic packets because this bread has antimycotic (anti-mould) chemical preservatives, such as calcium propionate). Make just enough bread for the day. Whilst pre-sliced bread is convenient, it perishes quicker due to a greater exposed area. Refrigerating bread does retard mould but actually makes it stale quicker, six times faster than at room temperature! (through "starch retrogadation") It is thus not an "intermediate step" between being at room temperature and freezing. The old way of keeping it in a cloth bag in a bread tin is better, but if over two days old, freeze the sliced bread and toast or warm slices in a toaster on demand.[43] Remember that mould is present long before it is visible to the naked eye, and that mould is the physical precursor to cancer, as we shall see.

Regarding the influence of blood type determining your diet, various studies have yielded contradictory results. In my personal case, and for those under my care, I have found some relevance but, again, personal observation and kinesiological testing[44] prove that each individual varies to a greater or lesser extent from the "norm" in a unique way.

Whatever your specific dietary requirements, real food is natural, not processed, with no synthetic inputs used in its production, or subsequently added to it, for whatever reason.

Having avoided chemicals, processed "food", and synthetic preservatives, colourants, aromas, stabilizers, and other chemical additives, you need to find what works best for you.

Some people are naturally in touch with their body and its optimal nutritional requirements. However, most people have become so out of touch with their bodies, that instead of being intuitively attracted to healthy foods, they are instead addicted to sugars, processed foods, and junk foods. Big junk "food" franchises have ways to addict consumers psychologically through (often subliminal) advertising, and physiologically by adding addictive chemicals, including sugar, harmful oils and (processed) salt. A cursive investigation into the junk "food" industry [45] will make anyone with integrity and self-respect who is not irrevocably addicted to it refuse to eat it again. Furthermore, if you believe (as an increasing number of people do, on the basis that the main constituent of meat is water-explanation later) that by eating meat you absorb the suffering of the animal, remember that one "Mac" patty may have the meat of 1000 animals from five continents. Assuming that we are 'designed' to absorb the suffering of one humanely raised and slaughtered animal, on traditionally rare occasions, what happens when we in essence repeatedly eat thousands (of cruelly raised cattle) at a time?[46]

It is disturbing to see that nearly all guides for healthy, alkaline blood and cancer prevention urge people to eat foods which are themselves alkaline. Paradoxically, eating overly alkaline foods may lead to an acidic system, instead of an alkaline one, and in addition may lead to other problems such as osteoporosis,, vascular plaque, etc. Why? Because much of our digestion needs our stomach to be highly acidic, with a pH of between one and three. If we eat overly alkaline food, we lose the ability to absorb such vital minerals as calcium and magnesium which, besides being nutritive in themselves and essential for our skeletal and bodily function, alkalize the body. This is particularly important as we age, as our stomach becomes less acidic.

That is why it is essential to differentiate between alkaline *food,* and alkaline *forming* or *alkalizing* food. It is also why mineral supplementation alone for osteoporosis may not only be unhelpful, but may cause further problems; and why people showing symptoms of mineral deficiencies may well develop vascular plaque despite low cholesterol counts, and stones in their gall bladder and kidneys of the very minerals their system lacks! To get calcium and other salts out of our blood (and thus kidneys) and into our bones where they should be, we need sufficient vitamin D and K_2.

Think of your stomach as the biochemical processor that it is. The acidity or alkalinity of your body depends not on the pH of your food you eat, but the result of its reaction with the hydrochloric acid in your stomach. Luckily, you don't have to be an expert chemist to understand the chemical reactions with everything you eat, provided you know that vegetables, particularly when organic, and especially when raw, are alkalizing. (Except for tomatoes which must be well ripened and aubergine which must be eaten in moderation, well cooked and preferably 'debittered' with coarse salt before cooking) Whilst peeled potatoes are fattening, the peel of the unpeeled potatoe contains an enzyme which breaks down the starch, making this a particularly nutritious vegetable in moderation. Never eat the peel separately, as is served in some junkfood outlets.

Particularly useful alkalizers are the paradoxically acidic lemon, grapefruit and cider vinegar.

It is thus essential that at least 70% of your food intake, preferably 80%, should be vegetables, and an ideal way of starting the day is with grapefruit, or at least half a lemon of juice on your food during the course of the day. Additional cider vinegar or lemon to alkalize an acidic system should theoretically not be necessary, though in practice our modern lifestyles tend to acidify most of us, to a greater or lesser extent, so check your system acidity (in urine)! (If you can get small quantities of litmus paper this is much cheaper than urine analysis sticks)

If you have found that you are not in optimal physical or psychological form, or you are attracted to unhealthy fare, you need help, redirection, and reprogramming. (Not medicines to mask the symptoms, i.e. the messengers of unhealthy living!) Your life, or at least the quality of it, literally depends on it! Find a dietician or therapist who preferably works with kinesiology.[47] Your body, not your head (what you think), or what anybody else (including "experts") think, always knows best, and applied muscle testing kinesiology is a technique of listening to what your body says. To determine what is right for you is a matter of high priority. That means right away! Should you wish to approach me for this, I have also helped many people remotely, also using kinesiology during my Skype personal consultations. Whilst most people who have approached me have been those already suffering with cancer, thankfully an increasing number is not, as more people realise that prevention (knowledge and awareness in action) is so much better than cure.

So much for natural food. Commercial farming, not only in animals but also agriculture, is the biggest culprit of environmental destruction, clearing vast tracts of forests, grasslands, and other biodiverse natural habitats to plant a single crop (monoculture).

A single plant grown in vast quantities, continuously, encourages the proliferation of organisms that eat it, as life forms naturally multiply according to the availability of food and sustenance. This is Nature's way of trying to restore environmental, ecological balance. Commercial, monocultural farmers then respond with toxic chemical poisons that have polluted land, water, and air over the entire biosphere.

The malignant mindset of monoculture (exactly analogous to the cancerous "unchecked cellular monoculture" in people) also causes farmers to poison and exterminate any organism which may eat crops, including the caterpillars that are the pupae of butterflies, essential for pollination of natural and agricultural plants alike. This also poisons insects other than those targeted, notably bees, as well as birds and other animals, their natural predators which, in a natural, un-poisoned environment, are all kept in perfect balance, in a dynamic and ever-evolving equilibrium (again, directly analogous to a healthy human or animal body).

Not even penguins in the South Pole can escape the poisoning, and are dying off as DDT (still widely used, although supposedly banned many years ago as it is not biodegradable) makes their egg shells too weak, so that chicks never develop to hatching maturity. Mid-ocean fish are also affected, becoming hermaphroditic, sterile and prone to cancers from manmade toxins and synthetic, hormone-laden sewage from women on the contraceptive pill, "HRT" and from livestock.

Our own drinking water is also contaminated; yes, municipal water is filtered and processed, supposedly fit for drinking, and in most places, tap water won't have you doubling over with typhoid or some other terrible disease. However, it is precisely because its toxicity is not immediately noticed that it is even more dangerous. The very agent which is usually used to "purify" water, chlorine, destroys water's life-giving qualities and is highly carcinogenic. In fact, according to the US Council on Environmental Quality: "Cancer risk among people drinking chlorinated water is *93% higher* than among those whose water does not contain chlorine."[48] Yet water in nearly all countries and US states is chlorinated and increasingly and deliberately fluoridated, despite *truly* independent studies (where the researchers have not been commissioned/paid by pharma companies, government or any other group with vested interests) proving the harmful (including carcinogenic) properties of both.

We are told that chlorination is necessary to purify water when far better processes, with health-giving, rather than health-destroying effects, exist, including ultra-violet irradiation and ozone treatment, as is done in Switzerland and some parts of France and Germany.[49] Peroxide and ionic silver are used in commercial airlines, spacecraft and by outdoor enthusiasts.[50]
Drinking plastic-bottled water does not solve the problem and may even worsen it. If at any time between bottling and drinking, the bottle is exposed to extreme temperatures, sunlight or even fluorescent lighting, your water will be contaminated with carcinogenic chlorinated compounds (such as PBA and phthalates) and other xenoestrogens (synthetic oestrogens (UK) or estrogens (USA)).[51] In addition, very few of these plastic bottles are being recycled, at a catastrophic environmental cost. If you "must" drink plastic bottled water, ensure that it is "still", not carbonated, with a pH at 6.8-7.4, ideally pH 7, (neutral, neither acid or alkaline) and that it is low on sodium and as close as possible to zero in fluoride. Remember to please ensure that the emptied bottle is then deposited in the recycling bin. I have been horrified to see water in upmarket shops with a pH as low as 4.5! Never freeze, boil, or microwave water in the plastic bottle as this considerably increases the water contamination, as stated by Dr Edward Fujimoto, in an article erroneously attributed to

'John' Hopkins University, and distributed by the Walter Reed Army Medical Center.[52]

If you want to take water with you for outdoor activities, use rigid acrylic, not PVC or soft, flexible bottles. An easy test is to open the lid of a new water bottle and sniff it. If it has a strong "plasticky" smell, don't buy it, as this toxic gas permeates your water, and do the next person the favour by passing on this advice.

While you, with every good intention, may do what you can to lessen your negative impact on the water supply, you unfortunately still need a water purifier. The water purifier must be one that removes the heavy metals, organic pollutants, hormones, fluoride, chlorine, and even radiation without removing essential natural mineral trace elements, notably calcium, magnesium and potassium, that would occur in a clean aquifer (underground water or spring). Reverse osmotic filters do a job of removing just about everything but H2O from the water. However, this water, stripped of all natural minerals, becomes acidic, and also causes beneficial minerals to leach out of your body[53] by osmosis, leaving you with serious mineral deficiencies, and vulnerable to a host of illnesses including cancer, due to its acidity, furthered through loss of alkalizing and mineralizing salts.

So unless your reverse osmosis purifier subsequently replaces these minerals (as some do), never drink reverse osmosis, distilled, or rain water (even if it is relatively unpolluted). If this is your only water supply, chew a dolomite or calcium/magnesium tablet with it, as this somewhat replicates the dolomitic and trace element-rich rock through which ground water flows. (Calcium and magnesium are synergistic in the body, the one facilitating the absorption of the other, and both are alkalizing).

I have selected the following water purifiers[54] as the best, in terms of quality, value for money, aesthetics, reliability, and after-sales service, and in my thoroughly researched opinion, by far the best value for money. Water is life, unless it is contaminated. And typical municipal water is badly contaminated. You need a *good, affordable* water purifier!

As chlorine also deoxygenates water, 'reoxygenate' your water either with an ozonizer or with a drop of **food grade** hydrogen peroxide (for 35%H_2O_2 a drop per glass or 4-5 drops per quart-litre will reogygenate water; read more on H_2O_2 on p 69.

But it doesn't end there. We ingest chlorine through the skin and inhalation (e.g., when bathing; Dr Coldwell refers to a shower as a "gas chamber") possibly more than through what we drink, making chlorine one of the top ten skin-absorbed carcinogens, as outlined in a single-paged, internationally researched document by ecosmartusa.com.[55] For this reason, you can get shower tap/faucet or entire home water purifiers here too[54] For the same reason, swimming in relatively unpolluted seawater is much healthier than swimming in a chlorinated pool, especially an indoor one, where the air is also permeated with chlorine fumes. If you have a pool, look into a salt water system. The chlorine in sodium chloride/salt is bound and thus not toxic as in normally chlorinated pools

Returning to farming, modern agriculture pollutes more, and has a far bigger carbon footprint,and is more environmentally destructive than all other industries put together. Ironically, people living in the country but near commercial farms are far more prone to environmentally induced illnesses than city dwellers, especially cancer from insecticide, herbicide, and other toxic sprays, as you can easily ascertain on the internet, starting here.[56] Most agricultural poisons do not simply "wash off" fruit and vegetables. They are "systemic", which means that the toxins are absorbed into the "flesh" of fruit and vegetables we eat.[57] In the case of GMOs, the toxin is also in the plant DNA itself. Furthermore, the nutritional value of produce from commercial farms is also diminished.[58] Especially so, hydroponically grown food (not to be confused with organic pescaponics/aquaponics). The hydroponic medium is a purely synthetic chemical cocktail which cannot possibly replicate the benefits of natural, micro-organism-based organic agriculture, even if all the necessary minerals are technically present.

Commercial farmers are fully aware of both the toxicity and abysmal nutritional value of their produce, which is why many have a small veggie patch near their house for their own needs.

Healthy soil, where a patch may still be found, is so rich in life as to have more micro-organisms in it than there are in the whole world above the soil.[59] This incredible living synergy is what feeds a healthy plant that provides vital (meaning "full of life"), nutritious food.

The reason for the extremely low nutritional value of commercial crops is that in order to grow the same crop continuously on vast tracts of land, and in order to maximize short-term profit, farmers are using synthetic fertilizers made of unnatural salts and petroleum extracts. These chemicals salinate (with salts of potassium, phosphorous etc), poison and destroy the ecology of the soil, necessitating more and more fertilizer each year. The destruction of the soil ecology also deprives the plant, and therefore us, of a myriad of micronutrients and trace elements *essential* to health, in organic form (which cannot be replicated inorganically) made available to plants only by micro-organisms in a healthy soil environment. Water resources are also contaminated by agricultural chemicals, and more precious water is needed to water crops due to increased soil salinity drawing water from plants through osmosis. This also results in less oxygen intake by roots. The resultant crop may look good but it is nutritionally deficient, tasteless and life-energy-deficient, as shown by Kirlian photography.[60]

We are also losing natural biodiversity (mainly due to habitat loss and pollution) and agricultural biodiversity at a terrifying rate as a few hybrids and GMOs are promoted to the exclusion of our original natural diverse wealth of "heirloom" food crop varieties. This is clearly not for the consumer's benefit, but to yield maximum profit to the seed and agri-chemical suppliers (such as Monsanto, Syngenta, and Du Pont), and consistent size, shape and longer shelf life for the supermarkets. Keep in mind that often the more nutritious, potent, and vibrant something is (i.e. connected to the natural cycle of life), the faster it then decays. Conversely, the more artificial or lifeless it is (i.e. removed from the lifecycle), the longer it takes to decompose back into its constituent elements. Furthermore, we have the chemicals which are sprayed onto harvested vegetables to enhance their aroma, make them look shinier and more attractive, crispier, etc, as well as further increasing shelf life.

Anybody eating nutritionally deficient, poisoned "food" is compromising their health, whilst supporting the industries that make it, and compromising the health of our environment.

Any effort to positively influence our economy to serve us and the environment, instead of these industries, is an effort to help reverse an economic cancer to which we have sold our souls. The Internet has enabled us all to be part-time activists through petitions and blogs, informing us of public meetings, networking opportunities, boycotts of harmful food, and active support of healthy produce, people, initiatives and other proactive actions.

Support local small farm markets, especially organic farm markets, an all-round healthy choice, not least of which is the personal trusting relationship created with the farmer. Our buying power, boycotting companies that disrespect our health and the wellbeing of animals and the planet, and purposefully buying from health-conscious companies that also treat staff humanely, are the instruments at our disposal for positive change in our lives, for our planet, and for the future. Never underestimate your power to significantly transform personal and mass consciousness.

It is frightening how "removed from life" we have become. Given the choice, animals will never eat commercial non-organic produce. In supermarkets, rats just love the organic section, if there is one, and totally ignore the other produce. A friend's rabbit ravenously devoured carrot tops from my vegetable garden. However when offered carrot tops from the supermarket, the bunny turned her nose up at them.[61] We eat most of our carrot tops as they are tasty, rich in fibre and very nutritious – carrots being a member of the parsley family. You just need to cut them up into short lengths to avoid choking on the fibre (as with parsley stalk).

The advent of hybrids means that the farmer or home gardener cannot harvest seed from his or her crop, as the next generation of crop would be indeterminable, inconsistent and almost certainly inferior. "Heirloom" or "purebred" traditional seeds are 100% "true to form" and more nutritious, bearing in mind that hybrids are commercially hybridised with patent rights and control over supply, with the profit motive (not your health), in mind. But hybridisation, whilst practiced deliberately, itself is not "unnatural", in the sense that different varieties/races of the same species, whether wheat or humans can, if in close proximity, naturally hybridise.

However, the most shocking terror attack on our health is the advent of so called "genetically modified (the aforementioned misleading euphemism for genetically mutated) organisms", or "GMOs", of all sorts, including and especially food crops and animals.[62] Companies such as Monsanto and Syngenta splice DNA belonging to completely different types of organisms into the DNA of plants and livestock. For instance, firefly DNA is spliced into tobacco and human genes into rice, the latter one may argue, effectively making us cannibals.[63] The reason offered to justify this is that in order to feed the world's population, we need to "modify" plants for higher yields, insect resistance, better shelf life and added nutrients etc. However, even where more nutrients are spliced into a plant's genes, they are not available to, or assimilated by, animals or humans that eat these crops. I have heard that human genes are now being spliced into a range of new genetically mutated animals for human consumption. How do you feel about being related to that pig you are intending to eat?

In truth, more than enough food is being produced, but our "civilization" values profit maximization higher (by dumping millions of tons of "excess" food annually) and also would rather allocate funds to global genocide via the arms industry rather than use them to distribute food to our starving brethren. The Borgen Project, along with numerous other analysts, cites the annual cost of ending world hunger (based on U.N. data) at $30billion, against the $737billion annual U.S.A military spending.[64]

Journalist Anthony Gucciardi also points out that eliminating world hunger would not simply be a philanthropic act but would all but eliminate illegal immigration and provide more economic fodder (return on investment), in terms of both productivity and consumption, for the consumerist, war-mongering multinationals and their governments.[65] A win-win situation.

A major reason for genetic "modification" is patently obvious (pun intended), as recent history has proven beyond any doubt whatsoever – (patented GMO's[66]). The purpose is to steal from humanity our food and sustenance by owning patent rights to seeds, animals and life forms in order to own and control all our food and other life forms, thereby creating artificial scarcity, and in "playing God", controlling life on the planet and owning our food, which we would have to buy from them or starve. In essence, "owning" the planet and all humanity. They've even patented human breast milk! (I did not believe this until I saw numerous references from various sources, including the mass media).[67]

As for cow's milk, Monsanto's recombinant Bovine Growth Hormone (rBGH) is poisoning cows, their meat, and especially their milk which, when consumed, far from preventing osteoporosis, worsens it and is strongly linked to cancer, especially breast cancer, and respiratory, circulatory, and other conditions. Government, the legal system and the media are all doing their best to misinform us in this regard.[68]

GM crops are NOT increasing yield, as we have been (mis) informed. In fact, they're doing the opposite,[69] and the assault of GM is worldwide. The "green revolution" experiment in India, in which GMOs latterly played a major role, resulted in an unprecedented famine, environmental destruction and bankruptcy due to unaffordably high-priced seeds, especially as farmers could no longer keep seeds from the previous season, as Man has done from time immemorial, due to purposely engineered sterile crops from "terminator seeds", forcing the farmer to keep buying seeds every season.

Unaffordable (to small farmers) expensive toxic chemicals needed for GMO crops are also part of the GMO "package deal". Record low crop yields resulted and even those who had sufficient food often fell sick, many of whom died from the sickening and carcinogenic nature of GMOs.[70]

How can you be healthy eating sterile, chemically grown and treated, genetically mutated grains, fruit and vegetables? For a start, at the most basic level, your whole internal flora and digestive system is disturbed. Studies have shown how GM foods can cause mutations or abnormalities in mammalian genetic code (in RNA and DNA), as conceded in two artcles in the U.S government health website, [62b, 68a] Interesting findings have also shown how olive oil can neutralize this harmful effect.[71]

Financial ruin, health disasters, starvation and suicides have proven to be the legacy of GMOs. To recover, India then literally had no option but to embark on an "organic revolution" and supplemented ancient wisdom with modern science in a way respectful to Nature, successfully producing a record crop, both in quantity and quality, resulting in a sharp drop in deaths and illnesses due to the improved health of her citizens.[72]

Right now in South Africa, almost all maize (US corn), the staple diet of most, especially poorer black South Africans and to a lesser extent, Afrikaners, is by design or contamination,GMO. Farm workers are dying from the maize they produce and eat, as one of thousands of examples of sickness and death from people and animals consuming GM foods, mainly soy and maize worldwide.[73] I am convinced that many deaths attributed to AIDS, particularly in South Africa, are in truth due to immune system collapse through GM "food", and general poor nutrition, making people vulnerable, often mortally, to many opportunistic illnesses. This genocidal selective poisoning of the black people of South Africa through GM is actively promoted by the supposedly "affirmative action" black government of the country, in the same way that the genocidal "Greek government" is, according to my dear and internationally celebrated friend Dr Mouroutis,[74] actively promoting the highly carcinogenic HPV vaccines not only to little prepubescent girls, but also little boys at the time of writing (with the ludicrous "justification" that they may become homosexual and that excluding all little boys would thus be "politically incorrect"!) [75]

Another GMO trick is to make food crops "Roundup Ready"

(i.e. resistant to this Monsanto herbicide) and insect resistant. That means that crops, instead of being killed by the weed killer, store the Roundup herbicide poison antidote (glyphosate) in their DNA. In addition, they are now also too poisonous for insects and other animals to eat. Contrary to the claims made by the GM companies, this toxicity does not "wear off" after harvest, as it is genetic. The only animals ignorant, "out of touch" and foolish enough to eat these crops out of choice are … you guessed it: modern humans. As a result, millions of people all over the world are becoming "mysteriously" ill, infertile and dying horrific early deaths, mainly presenting as cancer, amongst other illnesses.[76]

GM food is DNA-mutated food. The evidence against it, not in theory, but in tragic experience, is far beyond debate. However, if you are still not convinced, by all means do your own research, whilst keeping in mind that there is tremendous misinformation out there, mostly by "independent studies" commissioned by "the authorities" (read: puppets of vested interest, food-pirating multinationals). So don't be swayed by assertions and ridicule; check out the hard facts and use your brains; reason over emotional seduction. Remember Plutarch's admonition: "Your brain is not a receptacle waiting to be filled, but a Fire waiting to be lit."

Another problem is that GMOs are everywhere—in nearly all our processed food, 98% of soy, unspecified "vegetable oils", normally canola oil (which even before it was "modified" was never fit for consumption) and unnamed "starches". Investigating "GM" fully is obviously beyond this reference. However, this basic awareness is essential to any cancer prevention initiative. Consult a helpful guide, out of many available.[77]

In 2013, U.S. President Obama signed the "Monsanto Protection Act", the first time a government has ever signed a law giving a private business *carte blanche* to do what it wants and be effectively above the law, in blatant violation of human rights enshrined in the Constitution. Shortly thereafter the European Union installed GMOs in Europe against the wishes of the population and their national governments, whilst some relatively independent countries elsewhere hold out.[78] At the same time, President Putin of Russia banned GMO cultivation

60 The TRUTH about CANCER

and importation in Russia, for health and environmental reasons, including the obliteration of bees and health reasons, including cancer and, according to a report, threatened to go to war on the issue. "If you don't stop Monsanto, we will!"[79] This historically redefines our understandings of friends and enemies, transcending cancerous "us and them, divide and rule" tactics of national and political divisions, as we enter a new era where human values must and will once again prevail in the face of the aspirations of a one-world tyranny introduced using divide-and-rule tactics, amongst others. Russia is now dedicated to become GM &vaccination free, and the world's biggest exporter of not only GM free, but organic foods, with poor people being given land to this end. (the total opposite to policies in the "West", where mutlinational tyrants increasingly undermine health and monopolise the economy)

The good news is that, despite the above, and the fact that Monsanto has purchased Blackwater, the world's biggest mercenary army, public opinion is putting increasing pressure on them, particularly in Europe (despite legislation) and Argentina, where a partially built multimillion-dollar facility was suspended due to public opposition[80] until the government made a sudden, brutal about-turn against the wishes of the population, (I "wonder" why?) but with the latter winning out in the end due to the heroic commitment of many.

Besides decreasing yield, poisoning, patenting and monopolising life forms and food, the full story on the ecologically and economically disastrous effects of GMOs is beyond the purview of this book, but hopefully the point is clear: don't eat GM products or anything containing GMOs if you can help it, and support all initiatives for good, clean, honest food, and the *legible* labelling of any foods that deviate in any way from this.[81]

You, I and humanity have the key and the responsibility to restoring health to ourselves and the world. It is impossible to separate the individual from the whole. My writing this book is no less therapeutic to me writing it than it is to you reading and applying it; and your sharing it, and giving copies away to others, is likewise similarly therapeutic to you.

We all simply need to go back to real food – pure, fresh, organic produce. Avoid acid-forming carbonated and chemical cool drinks (especially "energy drinks"), meat, white flour, sugar, and excesses of dairy, tea, coffee, alcohol and processed/junk "food" in general. Drinking sufficient clean water, eating at least 70% (preferably 80%) vegetables of all types and colours, organic if available (mostly raw if you can), plus two or three fruits a day, and sufficient water (p64) is a general guideline for a healthy, alkaline system.

It is alarming to see the extent of tyranny in the U.S., which has, in some states, led to the prohibition of collecting rain water, which would otherwise be lost, and growing your own vegetables. Those communities affected must get together to reverse this tyrannical trend, and not be shy to call upon the rest of the world for support. The support is there, and only a few clicks away!

Finally, it would be remiss of me to not mention the importance of balancing our omega oil intake. With modern diets, we are consuming, according to oncologist Dr Phil Spiess, a ratio of 25:1 omega 6 to omega 3 oils, instead of the ideal 1:1 ratio. The US government Health site quotes research showing that the lower the ratio, the fewer the serious illnesses to which one is vulnerable.[82]

Dr Spiess also shows that eating fish and fish oil supplements is not the best way to restore this balance (he cites fish oils as being only 10% absorbed). My way of restoring omega 3 is by shredding a tablespoon full of flax/linseeds in a blender (quicker than grinding in a mortise and pestle) and sprinkling it on my morning muesli, already rich with a variety of nuts, dried and fresh fruit. If you do not want to do this daily, refrigerate an amount for, at most, a week in a dark container, as once crushed it quickly goes rancid. It is effective, cheap and I would say the most environmentally responsible way of omega 3 supplementation. If you don't feel up to doing this, Dr Spiess sells an omega 3 supplement which he argues convincingly is superior to other marine supplements.[83] Alternatively, you can use linseed oil capsules, or at least about a tablespoon of cold pressed Hemp/Cannabis oil (oil cold pressed from seed is legal everywhere and not euphoric) blended with about three times as much extra virgin olive oil (which is rich in the often overlooked omega 9) a day, preferably as a salad dressing. (Some people prefer the more expensive hemp oil capsules for convenience and avoidance of the "fishy" taste, but if mixed with olive oil as a salad dressing you won't notice it). Hemp oil also goes rancid fast, especially in a hot climate, so protect it from heat and light by keeping it refrigerated in a dark (green or brown) bottle, especially once opened.

Other foods generally recommended by many as anti-carcinogenic include lemon, cinnamon, turmeric (avoid if pregnant and seek advice if you have liver or kidney issues), pomegranates, broccoli, Brussels sprouts, kale and, to a lesser extent, cabbage (generally, the Brassica family of vegetables). These are all recommended by most informed health practitioners, one of whom is Dr Chakravarty.[84] Purely medicinal plants such as Sutherlandia (commonly known as cancer bush) and African potato are amongst an increasing number of plants found to prevent and combat cancer by acting against cancer-producing oestrogens. A more effective and direct approach to the leading carcinogenic effect of "oestrogen dominance" is discussed in the chapter dedicated to hormones.

When Jesus at the Last Supper offered the wine and bread as his blood and body, he was not conducting a transformational spell, nor did he intend to initiate a religious ritual. His message was clear and simple: What you eat and the frame of mind with which it was produced and prepared, especially when you eat it, together determine what you are. Your physical sustenance is a reflection of your spiritual sustenance. Indeed all faiths exhort us to honour our bodies as "temples of the divine" So if you are a Christian, you do not have to attend a special church ritual to commune with your Lord. Whether you are a Christian or not, it is up to you to honour your Creator and yourself to make every meal a "Holy Communion" in its fullest sense, and most definitely not hurriedly gobble trash. Whatever your decision, take responsibility for the consequences.

PRACTICAL

If you haven't done so already, check the ingredients of your processed food (canned, packed, dehydrated, prepared, frozen, etc.) for GM, known toxins or unknown ingredients.

1. If your diet is already a healthy one, pat yourself on the back. If not, commit to making a change in the right direction. It is better to make small commitments one at a time, and keep them, rather than an ambitious one that you can't and won't stick to. It is especially advised to start small with steady increments when you are preparing meals for uncooperative partners and families.

2. Buy food with awareness. Remember, organic food will cost more because it costs more to produce due to higher input costs, possibly lower short term yields and higher wastage rates and stocking costs due to shorter shelf life. Also, the product may be slightly insect eaten, and may even contain a couple of critters. This is actually a natural endorsement, because if insects are eating it, it must be good.

A 50% price premium on organic fruit and vegetables, generally speaking, is very reasonable. For ethically and organically raised meat, especially chicken, this can cost 100-200% more. One truly free-range chicken will require at least 10 times more space than a battery hen and about double the feed which is organic and relatively expensive, (and fowls take longer to grow without growth hormones), as it is free to run around, burning energy, whereas battery chickens are so tightly caged they cannot move, ensuring a disproportionally high (toxic) fat content, cutting feed cost, maximizing production, speeding up turnover and maximizing profit.

3. Be aware of what you eat, and take responsibility for your frame of mind whilst preparing and eating food. Eat with awareness and gratitude. Allocate at least one "formal communal/ion meal" a day with the family or household. If there seems "no time" for this, re-evaluate the priorities of the person with "no time".

4. Each one of us needs to become aware of, and be in touch with our own subtle body signals before they become severe, possibly irreversible and even deadly. Common indicators of acidity include arthritic/joint pains, gout, stiffness etc. Massage and physical activity, especially the former, are very important ways of achieving body awareness. If you are still relatively out of tune with your body, you could start off by testing your urine acidity.

5. For optimal health, drink water! It is recommended that you drink 1 litre (≈1 quart) of water daily for every 20kg (≈40lbs) of body mass, or about 1/20th of your body mass daily. You can drink 20% less on cold days when you are inactive, and 50% or more extra on very hot days when you are exerting yourself physically and perspiring copiously

If all the above recommended quantities for supplements and water intake sounds onerous, remember, they are guidelines. Unlike drug dosage, you don't need precise measurements, and after initial measuring, you will soon get the "feel" of the right amounts for you.

As for water intake, if your urine is markedly yellow (in the absence of other factors which may colour urine) you are not drinking enough water. Your urine stream should appear clear or almost clear.

6. If you have a garden, grow your own vegetables as much as possible. When I stayed in a flat, I planted veggies in pots. This is psychologically, spiritually, and nutritionally rewarding.

"He who sows the ground with care and diligence acquires greater stock of religious merit than he could gain by the repetition of ten thousand prayers."
– Zoroaster

2. OXYGEN, ACIDITY, & SUGAR

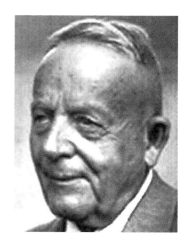

In 1931, Dr Otto Warburg won his first Nobel Prize for proving that cancer is caused by a lack of oxygen respiration in cells. He stated in an article titled "*The Prime Cause and Prevention of Cancer*" that "*the cause of cancer is no longer a mystery, we know it occurs*

whenever any cell is denied 60% of its oxygen requirements."

"Cancer, above all other diseases, has countless secondary causes. But, even for cancer, there is only one prime cause. Summarized in a few words, the prime cause of cancer is the replacement of the respiration of oxygen in normal body cells by a fermentation of sugar.

"All normal body cells meet their energy needs by respiration of oxygen, whereas cancer cells meet their energy needs in great part by fermentation.... deprive a cell of even 35% of its oxygen for 48 hours and it can become cancerous..... cancer cells cannot survive in the presence of high levels of oxygen, as found in an alkaline state."

– Dr Otto Warburg 1931, two time Nobel Laureate[85]

Due to the increasing burning of fossil fuels and the destruction of green habitat, particularly the planet's "lung," the Amazon Jungle, the killing of our oceans (even more oxygen is produced by ocean blue-green algae), and chopping down the tree in your own backyard, life-giving oxygen in the air has dropped over the years and is increasingly replaced by carbon dioxide, various toxic exhaust fumes and other man-made noxious gases.[86]

The main differences between healthy and cancer cells are oxygen deprivation and concomitant excessive relative acidity of the cancer cells. Most of our healthy cells are optimally neutral or slightly alkaline, and live off oxygen. By contrast, cancer cells are acidic, live primarily off a sugar-based fermentation process for energy and are actually "smothered", and even killed, by oxygen. Thus, oxygen can justifiably be said to be the prime selective cancer-cell killer and at the same time, life-giver and stimulant of healthy cells.

Causes of acidity leading to conditions favourable to fungus and cancer-cell proliferation are:
1. Lack of environmental oxygen in closed, badly ventilated environments.

2. Excess oestrogen (oestrogen dominance discussed under hormones,Chapter 5).
3. Excess CO2 from inefficient cellular discharge, shallow breathing and deliberate intake of sodas and fizzy drinks.
4. The pH of Coke® is 2.8, based on phosphoric acid. This causes osteoporosis, as bones, which are normally nitrified by phosphorus, attract this acid, together with the 8 teaspoons of sugar per can. Indeed, 'tis a concoction excellent for cleaning your toilet bowl, stripping rust, acidifying your system, dissolving teeth and bones. The pH of Red Bull® is 3.2. Remember that each number in the pH scale is ten times more acidic than the next. Vinegar has a pH of 3-3.5, but despite this, cider vinegar, lemon and grapefruit (not oranges) have a significant alkalizing effect on the body.
5. Stress, anger, resentment and anxiety cause shallow breathing resulting in incomplete CO2 expulsion, and insufficient oxygen intake, both causing acidity and compromising cellular and bodily function, as well as the secretion of acidic "fear chemicals," steroids, and hormones.
6. Exposure to electromagnetism from electrical and electronic sources.
7. Meat, especially from chemical-filled, stressed animals, typical of modern factory farms.
8. The "three white poisons", namely refined sugar, white wheat flour, and processed fine (cyanide, aluminium and other toxin containing)[87] table salt (not coarse sea or coarse mined salt which is essential in moderation).
9. Non-nutritive sweeteners such as Aspartame® (made from aspartic acid, phenylalanine and methanol), now marketed under deceptively "healthy sounding" names such as Nutrisweet® and Aminosweet® and made from the excrement of GM bacteria.[88]
10. Junk food synthesized from the aforementioned with the addition of animal fats and products, hydrogenated oil/fats, other "processed" oils, processed carbohydrates, various other synthetic chemicals and, increasingly, GMOs such as "corn or unspecified starch".
11. Modern diets with excessive harmful elements such as

fluoride, chlorine, and heavy metals such as cadmium, mercury and lead (plentiful in canned foods) all exacerbated by insufficient potassium and magnesium.[89]

12. Excess sugar is converted into lactic acid which cancer cells convert (back) to sugar, upon which they thrive.

13. Lack of adequate sleep and concomitant lack of melatonin, greatly exacerbated by watching monitors or TV screens, especially late at night and less than 20 minutes before sleeping. When one spends many night hours in artificial light, melatonin supplementation can be most helpful, both in falling asleep and in supplementing the loss of melatonin due to loss of darkness needed for our natural circadian rhythm. The more research is conducted in melatonin, the more significant its role appears to be to maintaining good health, youthfulness, a healthy head of hair and longevity, so I strongly maintain that loss of melatonin due to our modern lifestyle, with disturbed light and darkness cycle due to artificial lighting and lack of sleep, definitely warrants supplementation. More importantly, the American Cancer Society cites much research strongly suggesting that melatonin may well play a role in both the prevention and treatment of cancer on their site, www.cancer.org.[90] I thus strongly recommend this[91] **melatonin supplement**.

14. Most people are unaware that air conditioning, and most working environments rob us of oxygen, compromise our immune system, and make us vulnerable to infection in four ways: Firstly, the same recirculated air, with oxygen increasingly depleted, is increasingly replaced by carbon dioxide. Secondly, pathogens from everyone in the air-conditioned space are accumulated in every cycle, and even breed in the glass-fibre filters, exposing everybody to everybody else's pathogens. Thirdly, the air is positively ionized, so that even the little remaining oxygen is not efficiently absorbed, whereas in Nature it is negatively ionized for optimal oxygen uptake. The resultant drop of blood oxygen relative to hydrogen is also literally the formula for acidifying the body. Fourthly, the accumulation of toxins in the outgassing of photocopy machines and

printers, plastics, etc ("sick building syndrome") *which is discussed in more detail later.*

There appears to be much confusion between "good" oxygenation and "bad" oxidation, and the latter's connection to free-radicals, where oxygen plays a role in oxidizing, or the "rusting", of cells. Yes, the word oxygen itself is named after its potentially corrosive properties, coming from *"οξύ/oxy,"* which is Greek for acid, as it was once thought to be an essential ingredient in all acids, a claim which it lost to hydrogen. Hence, it is *lack* of oxygen which *causes acidity* in the body, due to a relative surplus of acid-forming hydrogen, whilst ample oxygen restores alkalinity, and conversely, alkalinity increases oxygen uptake.

This is a seemingly irreconcilable contradiction with respect to oxygen and oxidizing "free radicals"; a contradiction conveniently overlooked by mainstream medicine which can be reconciled when we understand, as "epigenetics" shows, that it is our predominant mind-state, together with the availability of calcium and magnesium, which determines whether this oxygen is used for our benefit (oxygenation) or the creation of "free radicals" (oxidation) which is effectively the biological equivalent to metal rusting.

How can you beneficially increase the oxygen in your blood in an oxygen starved environment?? Let's take a practical approach.

PRACTICAL (to increase oxygen levels and alkalize the body)

1. You've heard it before and you will keep hearing this: Exercise! This will be fully dealt with in the chapter on physicality.

2. Food-grade hydrogen peroxide (H_2O_2) bolsters our body oxygen content. Use *only* "food-grade" hydrogen peroxide (which comes only in 35% strength), not "regular" hydrogen peroxide, as this is contaminated with various poisonous chemicals. Put two to four drops of 35% food-grade hydrogen peroxide in a full water tumbler (approximately 250ml/8oz) of filtered water, twice a day, or 12 in a litre/quart jug, to be drunk over the course of the day. You can increase this gradually to a maximum of five drops to a full water tumbler (minimum 225ml/8oz). Higher dosages are gradually built up to 25 therapeutically, otherwise never exceed the above. Too much is dangerous![92] Handle 35% hydrogen peroxide with *extreme* care, as it is highly corrosive, flammable and even explosive. Mark it clearly (it looks like water) and keep it in the freezer (freezes at-3^{0}C) away from children and in a *childproof* bottle. Although "regular" (i.e. non-food grade) lower concentration peroxides are safer to store and handle, it cannot be overemphasized that these are toxic for internal use. If there is any possibility of ingestion by a child or anyone else, upon purchase dilute it 1:10 with distilled water and store in a brown bottle. The disadvantage of doing this is that it will degrade faster, depending on temperature and light exposure, but the ingestion of 35% concentration is extremely caustic and potentially fatal! Thus diluted, it is still dangerous to ingest, but around the strength of commercially available non food grade H_2O_2. Now just increase the dosage (drops) ten times, or analogous to the rate at which it is diluted. Hydrogen peroxide can be mixed with colloidal silver, enhacing the effects of both, but do not mix it with anything else, unless your chemistry knowledge justifies it.

3. Keep your system alkaline, using tests if necessary. The ideal midday urine pH is 6.8 to 7. Under that is not good, and under 6 under normal dietary conditions calls for urgent attention and it should leave you no doubt in terms of its signals or uncomfortable "symptoms", as mentioned.

Blood pH is around 7.34 to 7.4.Whilst the body as a whole may be acidic, the blood, in order to remain within the safe range will leach calcium from your bones, so that an acid system is not correctly diagnosable by blood pH, but by many indicators due to body acidity and/or calcium and/or magnesium deficiency. Calcium deficiency can manifest as muscle cramps, bone, tooth, nail and hair problems as well as insomnia, period problems or even late onset of puberty.[93] Excessive body alkalinity (alkalosis) seldom occurs naturally, happening only in such extreme situations as continuous vomiting, so dont worry about alkalosis if you follow, or even double alkalizing protocols mentioned here. The suggested protocols, based on an alkaline-forming diet, rectify acidity, returning you to the healthy pH neutral range. Adopt healthy habits and your body is quite capable of doing the "fine tuning"

4. To supplement with alkalizing magnesium (sorely lacking in most of us, and essential for a healthy cardiovascular system, the failure of which claims even more lives than cancer) and to balance it relative to acidifying sodium (excessive in modern diets, and consequently in a great majority of us), you can start adding incremental amounts of Epsom salts (magnesium sulphate) to the salt in your salt grinder. I know of a housewife who, fearing opposition from her family, does so covertly. Ensure that the container states that it is suitable for consumption, i.e. has no additional chemicals which could be added, for instance, to prevent clumping.

5. Buy only coarse sea or mined salt, never fine "table" salt, due to the harmful chemicals and additives in the latter. Keep in mind that "mined" salt was once, many years ago, sea salt, so provided there is no presence harmful of salts (such as cyanide or excessive fluoride) in the area it may be purer than "sea salt" due to absencee of man-made pollution. Drs Coldwell and Wallach's salt recommendations in two short videos will surprise many readers and are therefore recommended.[94]

6. Epsom Salts and bicarbonate of soda both alkalize you. Do not confuse bicarbonate of soda (aka sodium bicarbonate or baking soda) with the proprietary named Baking Powder® which contains various chemicals including aluminium. Bicarbonate of Soda is, according to Dr Tullio Simoncini (and as verified by many people who have "miraculously" recovered from a cancer "death sentence" imposed by their doctors), is uniquely fatal to cancer cells, over and above its alkalizing properties, and effectively used in his treatments using various protocols, depending on the cancer. Epsom salts replaces much needed magnesium which also facilitates uptake of calcium. When taking these, don't exceed a teaspoon per day in food or in water, keeping in mind that Epsom salts has laxative properties. Commercial alkalizing supplements are available (e.g. this one[95]), although I find recommendations in this book based on cheap readily available foods do the job just as well and are cheaper and more convenient. Bicarbonate of Soda is itself slightly alkaline and Epsom Salts slightly acidic, but both are alkalizing in the metabolism, the latter due to its magnesium (despite the fact that gardeners acidify the soil with it). However, for aforementioned reasons, I would rather use Bicarbonate of Soda "Trojan Horse" protocol as a treatment for cancer sufferers than for regular alkaline maintenance and Epsom Salts as a magnesium supplement, using the following as an alkalizing protocol instead.

7. A lemon a day eaten "as is", or squeezed in food, or half a grapefruit to start your day, or cider vinegar (1-2 tablespoons twice or thrice a day in a glass of water), all have a strongly alkalizing effect on the body. Cider vinegar is also a good source of potassium (another mineral sorely lacking in most of us). Some people drink cider vinegar in combination with bicarbonate of soda, but as the one is acidic and the other is alkaline, they react together, changing the therapeutic nature of both. More is not always better. One at a time! I believe Epsom salts should be used primarily as a magnesium supplement. Magnesium, as previously mentioned, is typically deficient in modern diets – with this deficiency also being a major cause of acidity.

8. Particularly if you are in a polluted or air-conditioned environment, get yourself an ionizer which creates negatively charged ozone, clearing the air (you can see black soot settling around it or in its filter) and "turbocharging" your oxygen uptake. Peruse information on ionizers, purifiers and recommendations.. If I can recommend one it will be posted on http://cancerfree.cf[96]

9. Finally, and most importantly, minimize, or eliminate, the intake of acid-forming processed foods and caffeine (coffee, tea) – although for most people one cup of medium-strength coffee or tea a day is quite acceptable. In fact, there are substantiated claims that, in such moderation, coffee, and to a lesser extent tea (especially anti-oxidising green tea) are anti-carcinogenic[97]. Beware however, as caffeine is highly addictive and you are far better off with no caffeine drinks than taking "energy" drinks, or being addicted to numerous cups of coffee daily.

Also eliminate all sodas, sugar and minimise alcohol, meat (especially processed meats) and dairy (lactic acid and casien, a standard wood glue), other than unadulterated full cream yoghurt. Increase your intake of vegetables and drink a lot of water. Remember that other liquids are no substitute for water and indeed, caffeine and alcohol drinks actually have a dehydrating affect, so that 200ml of coffee will deprive you of about 230ml of water and alcoholic drinks are even more dehydrating, this being a major cause of hangovers, as the brain is the first organ to be affected by dehydration.[103a] A most beneficial and really tasty home-made herbal infusion can be made of health-enhancing, cancer-preventing garden herbs including, in order of effectiveness, Cannabis leaves (if legal where you live; it is not psychoactive taken this way), origanum, sprigs of basil, rosemary and a drop of honey, stirred with a cinnamon stick. Even the pharma-medically committed U.S. National Library of Medicine acknowledges and praises the anti-carcinogenic properties of herbs and spices,[98a] and also gives an excellent, detailed account here.[98b] You can eat the leaves after drinking the infusion, or blend them beforehand into a powder which is filtered out or drunk in the infusion. To get more out of your herbs, you can dice them in a blender, but use immediately, as the smaller the herbs or spices are diced or ground, the quicker the essence, including flavour and aroma, is lost – especially if exposed to light and not stored in an airtight container. Dry your herbs for long-term storage to ensure an ongoing supply.

Keeping the leaves whole and in a sealed bottle in a dark, cool place will preserve them better than dicing them and putting them in a packet. Both cinnamon and cannabis are potent anti-carcinogens. Cannabis leaf infusion is not psychoactive due to its low THC content. Moreover, THC is not water soluble and needs to be heated to over 110^0C (235^0 F), above the boiling point of water, to be "decarboxylated" from THC acid to THC for its psychoactive effect and to be absorbed by a fat/oil (nonpolar) solvent. For an Indian Shiva worship ritual, psychoactive THC *tchai* is made by heating the Cannabis, particularly the flowers, in ghee (a butter-derived fat solvent) at a temperature high enough to dissolve and extract the THC before adding to the water. This video attests to extensive use of Cannabis in the Biblical era for food, medicine, clothing, rope, and mind altering ritual purposes, according to a senior rabbi and top academics. [98c]

You can vary the herbs according to availability, your tastes, and therapeutic needs. Have fun!

3. EMOTIONS

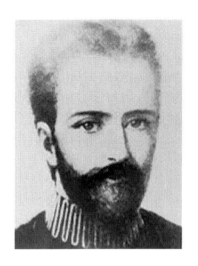

"It is the activity of our nerves, the flame of our desire, the acid of our fears, which daily consume our organism. He who succeeds in raising himself above his emotions, in suppressing in himself anger and the fear of illness, is capable of overcoming the attrition of the years and attaining an age at least double that at which men now die of old age. If the face of a man who is not tormented by his emotions should retain its youth, it would be no miracle."
– **Comte de St. Germain, 18th century alchemist, philosopher.**[99]

"It's scientifically proven that all illnesses are 84% based on stress and only 16% based on physical elements."
– **Dr Leonard Coldwell** [100]

Emotion may have its downside, as observed above, but it is nonetheless what moves us through life. A healthy person does not deny, but accepts and honours their emotions, whilst never indulging in them. E-motion is the driving force, and reason the faculty which directs it. That is why the Hindu elephant-god Ganesh has two tusks: one represents reason, which is intact, while the other, representing emotion, is broken, thus symbolically exhorting the temperance of emotion by reason.

Passion and emotion are very powerful. If strong and undirected by reason, they cause endless trauma and possibly even death to you and, in this day, the world. Directed by reason balanced with an open mind, miracles occur. A prime example of this is the Golden Age of Ancient Greece where the prime values of reason, virtue and balance *in all things* channelled their passionate nature to produce a quantum shift in humanity, a worldview to which we urgently need to return to save ourselves and a world overwhelmed by the cancers of unbridled greed, materialism and blind fanaticism.

With the progress of cutting-edge science in epigenetics, we are learning how denied or indulged emotions, and unquestioned, often unconscious beliefs, are increasingly being found to be the *prime source of health or illness,* especially cancer. Remember, we are energy beings (in scientific terminology) or souls/spiritual beings (in spiritual or religious terminology) expressing ourselves through physical form. We also know, however, that there is no "dividing line" between energy and matter, and that matter, which we experience and live through with our physical bodies, is merely the same energy in a lower frequency, so as to be experienced as a solid, or "tangible" state. In an analogous way, water transforms through various stages of its cycle as gas/steam/vapour, liquid and solid/ice. However in all its forms it is still water, and holds within it the same molecular structure, the same "additives", and the same memories, the latter a vital issue to which we shall later give the attention it deserves.

If we realise, then, that energy manifests as matter, and not the other way round, we acknowledge the primacy of energy, as expressed in our thoughts and emotions. A musician or sound technician will tell you how every note or frequency has "harmonics" in octave intervals of higher frequencies. A low note will always have harmonics of higher frequencies. These resonances/vibrations/frequencies create an energy field/ aura, which influences every cell in our body and, as a result, its function, shape, state of health, our external appearance and the internal structure and functioning of our organs. Most significantly, the energy field/aura complements, affects, and is affected by, our emotions in a positive feedback loop.

Some advanced mystics have mastered their energy state awareness to such an extent that they can drink poison with no ill effect, and I have witnessed self-inflicted severe body mutilations where the person did not experience fear or pain, and the wounds healed almost instantly, without a scar.

I am not advocating that you achieve or even aspire to such a state, let alone injure yourself. However, what I can demand of myself and appeal to you to do is that you *at the very least don't use your mind to make you sick*. This, too, is easier said than done, but the emotional basis of sound health (as explained in greater detail in my soon to be published book: "Living on Autopilot", (let me know if you would like a 'sneak preview') is the *most important* thing to which *everyone must give priority*, as the true foundation on which to build our lives and, as a consequence, to make the lives of others worth living and indeed joyous.

So that includes refusing to watch official news channels, letting go of negative friends, people and environments that "bring you down", and purposefully *being* love and radiating joy and allowing yourself to attract the same in your environment as a reflection of your own love and joy. This cannot be emphasized enough! There are many documented cases of people with "terminal" cancer recovering completely simply by undergoing a mindshift and by deliberate laughing (without "reason"). Is this not much easier, much more intelligent/sensible/rational, and a lot more fun? Is proactive health not far preferable to being a passive sponge of a negative environment waiting to get sick?[101]

When people discover that I don't have a TV set or read the newspapers, they often ask: "But how do you know what's going on?" To this I reply: "*That is exactly how I know what is going on; I won't let myself be drawn into the negativity, fear-mongering, victim consciousness and divide-and-rule lying tactics of a media designed to mislead and poison our minds and our lives. So I can therefore see things much more clearly.*"

Remember that, contrary to what you have been taught, health starts at the emotional level. The physical, whilst vital, is of a lower, subordinate resonance, and is thus secondary. Practice vigorous laughing often! Just as stress kills, laughter gives health and life! In addition to withdrawing harmful steroids and hormones in your body, and replacing them with healthful ones, it also gives you an oxygen surge and a unique deep internal massage where no therapist can ever reach![102]

The importance of laughter cannot possibly be overstated! It is *the* prerequisite for health, at the physical, mental and spiritual levels. Psychologically, laughter is the simplest, quickest and most fun way to achieve meaningful life transformation other than shock and pain, deep meditation or sincere prayer, second only to the responsible, guided use of certain mind-liberating or "soul-revealing" (psyche-delic) substances, to activate a mindshift to liberate us from being "stuck". Life is not static. It keeps on changing. So if you are stuck in a rut, you have a choice: either await a shocking event to shake you up, or choose to laugh *without any need to justify, or have a reason or "due cause"*, now! This is the most underrated *and* most powerful technique to stop being a reactive victim of circumstance and instead gaining mastery over (present) circumstance, with the intent of becoming a conscious, proactive creator of future circumstance.

You may have even heard of the anecdote of the man hospitalized to die of cancer decided that he may as well spend whatever money he had left to buy videos to "laugh himself off", only to fully recover!

(Now for your compulsory 5 minute laugh break! It's hard, initially, but once you choose to overcome your stuffy ego, believe me, it becomes easier!)

Have you done your laughing? I meant it! Do not read on until you have!

It is these interrelated abilities: to choose, and to laugh, which tangibly differentiate humans from other mammals. Laughter, especially laughter erupting from joy, which comes from within (as opposed to happiness, which comes from outside events, or circum-stance – i.e. things that "stand around" us), is indeed a spiritual connection to ourselves, to one another, and to our humanity. As the song says: "*Laugh, and the whole world laughs with you... the Sun comes shining through...*"

We all need to realise that Life *demands* its creation to

joyfully express its purpose in the world. Look at Nature. Any creature or organism that is not optimally expressing itself (as a unique instrument in the Grand Scheme) must be eliminated for the survival and optimal operation of the Whole. The clumsy predator starves, the weak antelope is taken by the lion, the feeble plant eaten by insects, and the miserable human succumbs to sickness. The animal and plant population benefit by the elimination of the sick and week, just like a single plant benefits when you prune the weak branches. The vines I did not prune died, while the pruned ones flourished. If you had an organization, would you also not retrench the negative elements, those which simply drain resources instead of making a positive contribution? Would your organization survive if you did not? If you have things that are outdated, broken, or constantly needing repair, is it not better to dispose of them, so that they may be recycled into something useful?

Adelle Davis (1904-74), the world renowned dietician who saved many thousands of lives by dietary prevention and curing of even "incurable" cancers, ironically died of cancer herself because, in her emphasis on diet, she forgot that state of mind is even more important. By contrast, George Burns, famous as a top comedian almost as much as his decadent junk food addiction, cheap plonk drinking, heavy smoking and "showcase unhealthy living style" worked well into his 90s and lived to 100, perfectly healthy till his death. While I am not advocating all aspects of his lifestyle, I do advocate his overriding philosophy of being perpetually joyful and spreading the joy around. Laughing out his strong "love of life" energy is also what magnetically attracted people to him throughout his life, and especially young ladies (full of the joys of their lives' "spring") in the last decade of his life after his wife died.

If you are going to eat healthy food out of fear, and not out of free will and joy for preferring living food over junk, you may be eating healthy food, but you are not eating healthily. Taking the Last Supper analogy a step further, when Jesus spoke about the bread and wine being his body and blood, He was not being macabre or making magic. He symbolically told us that *what* you eat is not as important as how; what emotional state and what associations and thoughts you have as you eat. The "physical food" that you take into your body represents and is energetically charged with, how and what you feed your mind.

It is *not true* that a Black Forest cake is tastier to eat than a carrot, and neither is the converse true. The truth is that food and everything else is only as enticing as the *meanings and feelings we (choose to or are conditioned to) associate with it.* Just as a man barely a hundred years ago was attracted to a pale and voluptuous woman, the "flavour" of our times is a slim, sun-tanned one, while a significant and growing minority of men may not be attracted to any woman, but to another man.

Constant media bombardment has all but obliterated reason and dumbed-down the good-sense of the masses, to the insane extent of convincing us that a certain beverage full of sugar, phosphoric acid, carbon dioxide and a myriad other chemicals "is Life!"; that processed GM meat patties in white flour buns is "the perfect meal"; and cakes and sweets symbolise the "sweet life" instead of the reality of diabetes.

We need a strong, disciplined mindset to reprogram our minds and redirect our emotions to enjoy real, wholesome, natural food. I grow the vegetables I eat and cannot contain my awe at seeing the seeds grow into the Living Miracle of Real Food. If you do not have the space or inclination to follow my example, then do the opposite. Go and see how the processed "food" you eat is made......*then* get your first bunch of seeds....

Occasionally, a dear friend will lovingly prepare you something that's "not so healthy" for you. As a naturopath friend of mine once maintained, the unavoidable *occasional* eating of a "not so healthy" meal outside your home environment may even "kickstart" your liver, and keep your immune system on its toes. This doesn't mean that you should use this as an excuse to compromise your (own) healthy eating habits, or drink that horrible brown fizzy drink. If your host does not have wine, or even fruit juice, you can always have the best drink; water!

Dr Emoto (I can't help but note the interesting similarity

between his Japanese name and the English word "emotion"), through his experiments with water, graphically and dramatically proved how even "clean" water is contaminated by "bad" thoughts, emotions, sentiments or feelings; and conversely, how "bad, dirty" water can be "healed" by loving energy. His books and colour plates comparing water crystals exposed to different music, ideas, emotions and thoughts, even names, are fascinating, making them wonderful coffee table books, both for their aesthetic appeal and as the perfect "ice breaker" ; exciting, yet meaningful conversation starters.

You do not need Dr Emoto's specialized equipment to witness these effects for yourself.

School experiments with rice and seedlings throughout the world have consistently proved the power of our thoughts, feelings and emotions to program water, which makes up 3/4 of our body, 8/10 of our brain, and the greater part of every living being; indeed the universal prime constituent and uniting factor of all life on Earth.[103]

Don't take my word for it. Try it yourself! Take two saucers with three bean seeds each (to exclude possibility of seed variances) and sprout them in wet cotton wool, paper or soil. On the one receptacle write, "Love", and on the other write something nasty (possibly a curse word you may use). Now place them where they receive the same amount of light. Every morning and every time you walk past them, pick them both up in turn and say the respective word, preferably but not necessarily passionately to each and check the differences over the next few weeks. You may also choose to have another similar receptacle of three beans which is totally ignored except for watering, as a "control".

This is a simple, fun and fascinating experiment for a family, school or other group. I also performed an experiment which Emoto recommends with brown rice, on my own, with my daughter and with various groups, with consistent results. After three months, the rice in the sealed jar with "hate" written on it was almost black, with a foul odour, whilst the other identical jar with "Love" written on it was off-white and fermented, with a pleasant sweet smell, as seen in this video.[104] Seeing is believing! But wait, what if the video is fraudulent? I *don't* want you to simply believe. I want you to *try* it, *experience* it and *know* it for yourself!

Now remember that water is the uniting element of all life forms, makes up over 3/4 of our planet's surface, of our body, about 80% of our brain and heart and around 90% of our blood. If "programmed" water has such a significant and measurable effect on non-human life forms, what can it do for us? This is the basis of homeopathy.[105]

On a "deeper" level, did you know that your pineal ("pine cone") gland, situated in the centre of the brain, considered by all major spiritual and religious traditions to be our spiritual-physical link, is a hollow gland, the inner surface of which is lined with the same rod and cone light receptors as your eyes, and filled with… pure water? What images could this "third eye" possibly be perceiving in the water? Is this a totally irrelevant natural anomaly, or an accessible and programmable phenomenon deserving its own book? What are your views on this?

For those of you who still underrate the importance of the psycho-emotional element to health, and need to see the stats to be convinced, it is worth noting that the countries with the highest incidence of cancer, i.e. Anglo-Teutonic cultures, while being the least environmentally polluted and the most health-food conscious, are nevertheless "emotionally tight", which tends to undo all the benefits of the former characteristics. Denmark tops the list, followed by Ireland, Australia and pristine New Zealand, with sparsely populated, forested Norway and Canada almost as bad as the world junk food capital, the U.S., in seventh place. Much poorer, densely populated and thus more polluted countries with much more challenging lifestyles, but with a more spontaneous and less stiff, more tolerant and compassionate take on life than the "cold and rigid" Anglo-Teutonic way, were way down the list. That more emotionally expressive women are slightly less prone to cancer, but increasingly more susceptible as they "masulinise" in seeking gender equality based on male standards would support this hypothesis.[106] So, a holiday to Cyprus, Greece or Cuba, besides being excellent destinations, have the unadvertised advantage of teaching us a "no-cancer" mentality! (In fairness, another differentiating characteristic of these "high incidence" countries is inordinately high dairy consumption. There is no conclusive study to prove which factor is more significant; though in my opinion, whilst not discounting the dangers of excessive dairy intake, especially as pasteurized, synthetic hormone laden cow's milk, I strongly believe that negative emotional factors (supressed emotions and harboured resentments) are by far the dominant culprits.

Bottom line: Honesty with yourself is a prerequisite to honesty with others. This in turn is a prerequisite to integrity (integrating and genuinely acknowledging all of your feelings and beliefs), which is the foundation for love, as opposed to a superficial "politeness and niceness" covering a cauldron of treacherous, cancerous thoughts. Honesty and integrity does require courage, and can hurt short term, but prevents the buildup of suppressed feelings which become toxic, (and eventually cancerous) thus liberating you and those you deal with for the benefit of all. ("The Truth shall set you Free" NT John 8:31).

Now, theory is all very well, but you have practical work before you move on. Knowledge of the head won't get you out of bed! Involve your Heart to Make a Start!

EMOTIONAL PRACTICAL – 1
Go through your friends/contact list. Seek out the most negative people you know. You know the ones I mean. Maybe you are one of them yourself. Are you? From your contact list find every person that is negative, crotchety and a pain in the nether regions. Delete them.

Is it a 10th of your contacts? A quarter? If it's over a third, be a bit concerned, for the more such people in your list, the more the evidence points to you being the type of person that you should avoid! You know the saying: "Like attracts like". Wealth coaches remind us that our wealth is the average of that of our five best friends. As I am not specifically a wealth coach, but an Overall Health Coach, I recommend that you seek out friends in all areas you would like to develop, for *mutual* benefit. Some may bring out your intellect, some your aspirations for material wealth, others can improve your golf game, your social contribution, and yet others, never to be underrated, your need for humour.

What do you get out of each friendship, and what do you put in? Friendship is never a one-way street. You may (to your credit and benefit) love the whole world unconditionally, but friendship is a selective, transactional as well as a transformational relationship. It is not a static relationship, but one which either evolves or regresses. Your choice of friends is an outward statement of your own identity, values and intent as to where you want to be, and/or where you want to take your life, in one specific way or another, or in general. Be aware, and keep assessing yourself through the friends you choose Just as the 'flu is contagious, a cancerous state of mind is even more so.

If you are presently a "rotten egg", that could mean throwing out your whole "rotten" social circle, and that it is time to get out there, *recreate yourself,* and by your new, purposefully, proactively joyful and positive demeanour, attract new friends – and a new *Life.* Do this before a turn in your health imposes this decision on you.

This is not easy. If you find it difficult, rest assured: getting out of a rut and challenging ourselves to become better people is difficult for me, for you and for us all, and the temptation from the false sense of security to "stay as we are" comes naturally and is so much easier. But amputation of the sick part is often needed for the greater good, and in some instances, such as gangrene (physical or psychic), it could even be the difference between life and death. If you have been, or decide to be, positive, generous, success-minded and joyful yourself, your pruning will be minimal and much less traumatic.

You may find that you are particularly reluctant to let go of a particular friend, as I have found. We had had an intimate relationship at one time and life circumstance separated us, but we had remained friends. What I have done in this situation is telephone her and tell her what I am doing, and that I would rather terminate the friendship with her than have negativity and hear moans and complaints. I choose any future interaction I partake in with anyone to be positive and empowering for both sides. I do not want to be guilty in partaking in her negativity, and neither do I accept negativity from anyone any more, irrespective of who they may be. I meant, and mean it.

Act now, before you read on. "Fire all the bad workers" in the business of your life, as if your life (or at least the quality of it) depends on it, which it does." As for the exception I made for my friend? Maybe I'm a bit of a sentimental wimp.... OK, I admit it; it would be dishonest of me to deny it and hypocritical of me to expect you to do otherwise, so if you do make an exception, make sure it's only to *one* person who *respects* you and in your *honest* opinion is likely to respond to your ultimatum. As an aside, the abovementioned person has since failed to meet my requirements, thus terminating our relationship. I thus lovingly give her the opportunity to learn and *become* the loving encouragement for which she depended on me. True love is tough, and contrary to common belief, not for "wimps" or those who choose weakness, avoidance, emotional attachment and its counterpart, blame.

Now close the book, and don't open it until you have purged your list.....

EMOTIONAL PRACTICAL – 2
Welcome back. How do you feel? Awesome! You have just plotted yourself the best course, with the best crew. Even a "skeleton crew" is better than a whole bunch of mutineers. However, the toughest challenge is yet to come! Your boat is still very low in the water, and the slightest breeze could be all it takes to sink you.

What can it be that's perilously weighing you down? You look around everywhere and you can't find it. But I can see it clearly.

Why? Because you are carrying it on your back – a sack full of grudges, fears and regrets. Maybe you have been carrying this bag for so long that you are no longer aware of it. Meanwhile you are all hunched up, and unbeknown to you, all your decisions, conscious and unconscious, are influenced by this misdirected energy. This bag is also the *primary hidden* cause of cancer according to my research, and that done by many top experts in the field. Dumping this alone, even if you do nothing else, minimizes or even eliminates your risk.

Now be honest. Real honesty has nothing to do with other people. That is secondary. You cannot be honest with anyone else unless you are honest with yourself, just as you cannot be faithful to anyone unless you are faithful to yourself. And you cannot love anyone unless you accept yourself and Be Love first. Who do you resent at this moment? Who in your past has stolen, cheated, betrayed, violated or harmed you in any way? How do you feel about them? Write down their names here, now, and next to them what they have done to you.

1 ....

2 ....

3 ....

Three will do for now. If you have more, revert to this exercise tomorrow and repeat it. I can't tell you how many to work on, and neither can you. Your body will tell you when you are sufficiently purged, as you will *literally* feel lighter and taller as you *physically* feel yourself freed of the weight.

Do you wish you could somehow get back at them? As long as you silently hold grudges against them, this poison is trapped within you, and has nowhere to go, as it cannot vent on the person you despise, who is blissfully unaware. It therefore quietly takes out its venom in the only way it can, contaminating, burdening and consuming your life, until something "happens", which could well be a heart attack or cancer.

Now be honest. Not with me, or with anyone else. Be honest

with yourself. Look at this list of names, one at a time. What other options do you have besides holding a grudge? Divorce? Legal action? Beating them up or killing them? Deflating their tyres? Would revenge in any way fix things? Would phoning them and telling them off? Seducing their spouse? Forgiving them? One option which is not open is forgetting about them, for if that were possible, you would have done that already and the only result was denial. So there is no way out. You need to commit to some action and you need to commit to it right away. No one is as dishonest as those who lie to themselves and none shall reap sterner punishment.

Now write a list of as many options for each of the three as your imagination will permit, without judging them, good or bad, childish or stupid, moral or immoral, predictable or unpredictable etc. The only criterion is whether it is possible for you.

1. ....
2. ....
3. ....
4. ....
5. ....
6. ....

1. ....
2. ....
3. ....
4. ....
5. ....
6. ....

1. ....
2. ....
3. ....
4. ....
5. ....
6. ....

Know that each course of action has consequences – for them, for you and, indirectly, for others. Then take action – one by one on those three people. Set yourself free. Whatever option you do take, be prepared to accept the consequences thereof. Everything has a price, and if we are pushed by our unbridled emotions, the price may well be far more than what it's worth. A shrewd investor, whether in money or emotions, must strive for the greatest benefit at the lowest cost. If, for instance, you choose to avenge your perceived transgressor, be prepared to accept that it is most unlikely that you will get away with it and the cost or consequences will be even worse, hounding you more than ever.

I do not favour or recommend vengeance, not because I am a "good person", but because I choose to take "response-ability" for whatever happens and whatever I do in my life. Reaction is a victim's unconscious, "kneejerk" inability to choose a response, to reclaim the power of "response-ability". I refuse to perceive myself as a victim or to empower anybody, under any circumstances, to deprive me of choice or to make me act in a way inconsistent with my ethics.

I also know that by being trapped, refusing to learn, not transcending or letting go of the past, the past will keep coming back to me, as its lifelong prisoner. What does a strong, passionate but misdirected energy do to the cells in your body? You now know!

If you go the way of vengeance, it is your choice and responsibility. You are empowering others to make you an eternal victim, and investing time, effort and energy of your life that will in no way improve, but poison it.

However, should you decide to forgive anyone, you are not doing it for them, or deciding based on whether you think *they* deserve it or not, but because *you* deserve to be free and to walk tall. This does not mean that you like them, that you will associate with them, or give them the opportunity to do it to you again.

In fact, by taking revenge, you entrench your victim mindset, and are far *more likely* to be hurt in a similar way by someone else than if you forgive and move on, not by denying, but having learned from the experience and now much the wiser. The Greek word for forgiveness, which profoundly illustrates the mechanism of forgiveness, is συν-χόρεση/syn-chorese, which literally means "together-fit", to integrate rather than resist, for "what you resist, persists". (CG Jung).

In fact, forgiving may paradoxically be the ultimate (albeit unwitting) revenge, as, having forgiven, you now take your energy back, re-centre yourself, focus and dedicate yourself to yourself, to be as joyful and successful as possible, while the other party, by choosing predatory behaviour, remains un-centred and squanders their energy outwardly and negatively.

In many families, communities, cultures, religions and nations, grudges and violent antagonism have followed many generations, very often long after the initial reason for antagonism was forgotten, whilst increasing exchanges of malice create a self-fulfilling belief of the evils of the "other" and thus the "justification" for intensifying the vicious cycle for generations to come.

The renowned statesman Nelson Mandela was no saint, in fact, far from it, but when he chose to forgive all the brutal wrongdoings perpetrated on his people and being imprisoned for the best 27 years of his life, said "Resentment is (like) drinking poison and hoping that your enemy dies."[107] It was due to his incredible commitment to forgiveness that he "miraculously" led South Africa from the inevitable bloody outcome of a country at war with itself, immortalizing him in the eyes of the world.

Precisely the same principles apply to you and your own life. Take response-ability for, and have mastery over the poison, before it kills you, and create a miracle out of it! Remember some of the most powerful cures are derived from the deliberate, altruistic and purposeful *transmutation* (not denial) of poisons, whether physical or emotional.

Now, if you really did this properly and sincerely, you will notice that you are feeling even lighter, taller, and breathing more deeply than before, delivering more precious oxygen to your cells which, as we know, is a major cancer preventative in itself. Over time you will notice that you are less stressed, more focused, more "in the moment" and have less of that nasty adrenaline and cortisol coursing through your veins, and more endorphins ("happy hormones"), putting you on the natural high that life intended for you.

But it gets even deeper, better and closer, … NEXT is the real clincher... But leave it for now… You are doing well! Allow yourself to integrate this forgiveness, to feel it literally in your heart for at least a day, before you read on…

EMOTIONAL PRACTICAL – 3

Welcome back! Did you have the courage and integrity to forgive? If not, try again, before we move on. This is essential!

Are we ready? Eliminate all distractions for at least 40 minutes, preferably the last hour before going to sleep. You have a sleeping partner? Invite your partner or family to do the same exercise at the same time (if you have not already done so for the previous exercises). If you honour yourself in the slightest you will doubtlessly switch off your communication devices and issue strict instructions that nobody is to disturb you for any reason other than mortal danger. Now that we have dealt with the issues that we have had with others, it's time to deal with the person the other three fingers were pointing at. Yes, it's your turn!

Below, write down at least three things/events you have never forgiven yourself for. It could well include allowing yourself to be betrayed by one or more of the person/s mentioned above.

1.

2.

3.
....

....

4.
....

....

....

You now have two options. The first is not forgiving yourself. The consequences of not forgiving yourself are even more dire than not forgiving others, because, in effect, you are constantly telling yourself that you are "bad", or the kind of person that makes these "stupid mistakes", an unshakable identification with everything you are desperate to avoid; punishing, avenging *yourself.* This inevitably results in you creating and attracting more such "mistakes" and misfortunes, whereas the Truth is that you were doing what you thought was best according to your knowledge and emotional development at that particular moment in the past (otherwise you would not have done it), and now you know different. You cannot hold onto and let go of something at the same time. Fear, guilt, regret, anger and anxiety cannot occupy the same place as forgiveness and love.

However, by forgiving yourself, you can learn, benefit from the experience, and let it go, so that next time you can make decisions based on what you have learnt.

Thus, we remember that emotions are not our enemy, to be resisted or denied, but need to be harmoniously tempered and directed with reason, as two sides of the same coin, and not as antagonists or polar opposites. We shall discover the final secret of achieving this before the end of this book.

Becoming victims to our emotions or masters in accepting and transcending them is probably the most profound decision we can ever make between cancer and radiant health, in the same way that we respond to any messenger who brings us important information (about ourselves) we may not like.

4. ELECTROMAGNETISM

"Sensitivity to electromagnetic radiation is the emerging health problem of the 21st century. It is imperative that health practitioners, governments, schools, and parents learn more about it. The human health stakes are significant."
– **Dr William Rea.**[108]

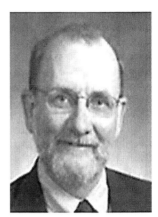

Everything visible or invisible, energy or matter, has its own vibratory resonance. Everything, including life and even death, is energy in vibration; and everything can be reduced to, or categorized as, a bundle of frequencies. The human race has its own frequency or vibration, as has every belief system and each one of us in turn have our own, unique personal vibration.

However, whilst the universe is composed of a perfect symphony of vibratory frequencies, electromagnetic and otherwise, the human race is generating and playing with electromagnetic fields without a clue as to their hidden immediate, medium and long-term consequences.

Most definitely, electromagnetic pollution,("e-smog") with trillions of bits of electromagnetic information continuously flowing through us, is happening for the first time (to the best of our knowledge) in recorded human history, and we thus have no precedent for knowing its long-term effects.

Sonograms have conclusively proven that cellphone radiation, commonly at a frequency of 19MHz in the U.S. and 18MHz in most other countries, has a definite impact on our brain, and double that impact on the brain of a child under 16, whose skull is thinner and whose brain is still developing.[109] Is it a coincidence that this frequency range, half that of a microwave oven, has been used as a secret weapon by the military?[110] Should we simply dismiss as "anecdotal" that brain cancers tend to be one of the faster growing types of cancer which "coincidentally" is more prevalent with people that spend more time speaking on cell phones? Even though cell phone radiation is reputedly "non ionizing"?

If you use a cellphone, it is best, wherever possible, to use it on speakerphone and second-best with Bluetooth® which has a less dangerous frequency and much lower power. But don't keep it permanently at your ear. See what Dr Sinatra and others[111] have to say about radiation, including cellphones, and do some of your own experimentation on cellphones, such as these.[112] The old corded earphone option is worst, as the cord amplifies radiation by acting as an antenna. Finally, the safety advantages of speakerphone with the privacy advantages of earphones can be achieved with tubephones, as explained here.[113]

Some Scandinavians prohibit child use of cellphones and many also keep their phones in an ankle holster, far from sensitive organs. Good idea. Alternatively, if one wears cargo trousers with many pockets, one could keep the phone in a lower pocket. Another advantage of these, if you live in a high-crime area, is that it is more difficult to pick-pocket from there.
The most dangerous place to keep it is in your underwear where you are inviting genital, prostate/uterine or breast cancer.

Don't share the same space as transmission antennae, whether they be cellphone, radio/TV, radar or any other electromagnetic transmission system. Many studies have proved the dramatically increased incidence of cancer for people that live or work within 100m (110 yards) of such antennae or high-tension electrical cables. Children are particularly vulnerable, and ironically schools are a place of preference for placing mobile communication transmitters. Sadly, many schools in poorer areas eagerly snap up what they see as a benevolent passive rental income from such a mast.[114]

At home or at work, connect to the internet, local network or printer by cord, rather than Wi-Fi. If you "have" to use Wi-Fi, try and keep at least about two paces from your router (i.e. install it away from your desk and bed) and switch it off when not in use. Some routers have a switch to switch Wi-Fi on or off whilst using the ethernet cord. Corded connections are in any case a faster and more efficient means of connecting to a router.[115]

Electromagnetic radiation is also emitted from all your electric and electronic devices, particularly computers and especially laptops and tablets where the processor is in or right under your hands, even on your lap. Laptop manufacturers warn you to keep their "laptops" off your lap, due to electromagnetic "burn," which makes your thighs bright red or blue, full of varicose veins, but worse, exposes you to the very real danger of reproductive system cancer which constitutes, generally, the highest incidence of cancer in both sexes.

There is no way we can prevent exposure to all, or even most radiation we are exposed to, but there are many ways we can limit it and/or transmute its effects. Either minimize exposure by avoiding electromagnetic apparatuses (which, for most of us, is impractical), or protect your children and yourself with electromagnetic neutralizers that don't eliminate electromagnetism, but modify it to a less dangerous form, placing them in various spots in your living area. Orgonite" devices of about grape fruit size can be ornamental and bought or made for living areas or placed near sources of radiation. We shall also look at much smaller , almost paper thin devices which   I use.

I distrust most products used for neutralizing radiation, so to help you to avoid getting caught, I direct you to [116] where you can acquire excellent radiation neutralizers, dependent on the nature of the electromagnetic field and the area you need to be covered. Alternatively make your own orgon devices[117]. There are also compact personal and equipment (cell and cordless phone, laptop computer, TV/monitor) radiation neutralizers I highly recommend the goods and services of the delightful and most helpful Dr Bindi in Europe, and Paulo Asaamora in the United States[118] I use their products on my cell phone, all my electronic devices , and on my electrical distribution board.

If you have allowed the electricity utility to install a dangerous "smart meter", (don't!) or if there is one in proximity, it is *essential* to have one of the the above people's devices installed near it.

However, do not rely just on getting "external fixits", essential though they may be for our modern electromagnetically crammed world. Be practical. If you watch TV and still have an old cathode ray tube (CRT) monitor or TV set, replace it with a new flat-screen one of any type. Or, better still, don't replace the TV! The radiation emanating from the cathode ray electron gun is deadly, not to mention the propaganda transmitted on TV that poisons your mind, or the unhealthy, high-pitched carrier wave. I know of a case where a young couple "mysteriously" lost their child to leukaemia.[119] The child's cot was near a wall on the other side of which was a CRT TV. If you are really attached to having TV and cannot afford to replace your old CRT TV, you definitely must have the back of it facing an outside wall and keep a distance of at least three, preferably five times the diagonal measurement of the screen away from it.[120]

If you use an electric blanket, unplug it before you enter your bed. Under no circumstances, no matter how tempting, must you ever sleep with it on. Space permitting, sleep 3 metres/10 feet or more away from any electric or electronic equipment, especially metal heating radiators.[121]

I must also mention that there is a view that magnetic fields from fridge magnets can be carcinogenic. I am not qualified to comment on this, but am not convinced, as these magnets are very weak, and once stuck on the metal door, very little magnetism radiates from the now closed system. By contrast, the fridge compressor motor and even the door use much stronger magnets, and if there should be any problem with magnetic or electromagnetic fields, it would be from here. However, over 100 years of refrigeration have yielded no scientific or anecdotal claims, or any evidence of harmful effects. I nonetheless make better use of my fridge/freezer door with a special "whiteboard" type surface, which I use as a daily inspiration, kitchen shopping, and meal planning board.[122]

Oh, and by the way, if you can cook with gas, it is not only cheaper and instantly responsive to your temperature adjustments, but healthier for electromagnetic reasons and interestingly, the food tastes better! Don't just believe me. Try it yourself! As for the metal induction stoves, I would stay way clear of them!

On an even more positive, green note, plants are known to be absorbers and neutralizers of harmful electromagnetism, as well as cleaning and energizing the air, providing oxygen and uplifting you psychologically. Cacti are low maintenance and particularly reputed for their absorption of electromagnetism, especially the Christmas cactus for the bedroom, as they also release oxygen at night, a time when most plants are in their oxygen absorbing cycle (it is also cat proof). Incidently, *feng shui* fans are opposed to having them indoors. I must admit, I also find prickly cacti rather unfriendly, but luckily there are other plants with the same benefits which grow well indoors. These include the African violet, all succulents, the spider plant *(Chlorophytum comosum)* and many more. Visit your local nursery for plants suitable for your local conditions for home and office.[123]

As for absorption of radiation, the recently late Dr Emoto particularly recommended the Cannabis plant, maintaining that it should be planted extensively around the damaged nuclear reactors in Japan due to its exceptionally powerful effect of absorbing and transmuting radiation.[124] This plant is already touted as a cancer preventer and treatment second to none, especially in the form of oil extract, and single most successful therapeutic remedy by many sources, from thousands of former cancer sufferers to top academics in Harvard University.[125]

Remember that buildings, particularly office buildings, also have a high concentration of plastics and synthetic materials which release carcinogenic "VOCs" (Volatile Organic Compounds), responsible for the notorious "sick building" syndrome, for which NASA has actively promoted the use of indoor plants as an effective antidote.[126] Despite this, wherever possible, keep printers and copiers (which emit toxic gases including carbon monoxide) near an open window or ventilation, never in a small, enclosed space.[127]

Please note that the term "organic" (other than in the context of food) unfortunately does not always equate to wholesome and health-giving, or even "natural". It means any compound based on carbon, including toxic paints, plastics, all petroleum products including the absorbent gel in tampons and diapers, "baby oil," "technical oil" used by physiotherapists, synthetic materials, insecticides, etc. (Yes, chuck out those nylon knickers, or at least keep them for those "special occasions"). You should not have synthetics against your skin, particularly your sensitive genital areas. [128] This is particularly problematic if a woman's pubic hair is shaved and there is direct skin contact restricting pheromone laden perspiration and evaporation on the one hand and on the other, closing the feminine aperture, not allowing it to "breathe", creating the ideal environment for anaerobic and partially anaerobic bacteria or fungi, resulting in cystitis, possibly leading to cancer in the female genital passage and organs. Another "underwear issue" is string or thong underwear, which draw faecal contamination to the female genitalia. If you insist on using these panties, dip the thong into colloidal silver before wearing.

Fluorescent lamps emit considerable radiation at close range, especially cheap no-name brands with a single "envelope" of white powder coating which increases the possibility of radiation leaking through tiny gaps in it. Should they accidentally be broken, you are exposed to mercury poisoning, both tactile and by inhalation. Do yourself and the environment a favour and replace these mercury-containing lamps, disposing of them properly, at your earliest convenience, for appropriate recycling, something seldom done. Replace them with either the old incandescent globe or, better still, the most economic LED lamps. Although the latter cost more initially, their lowest consumption and longest life, compared to both incandescent and fluorescent light fittings, makes them the cheapest, safest and most eco-friendly option in the medium to long run.[129]

Of course, this section would not be complete without

discussing microwave ovens. I refer you to some interesting articles and videos by experts in their field[130] and repeated experiments first done by schoolgirls[131] whereby a cup or pot of bean seeds are sprouted with cooled off water previously boiled in a kettle and similar container of beans are spouted with water from the same source but boiled in a microwave oven. The difference in growth is striking! I won't tell you more. Before you consult the reference, try it for yourself, and act according to *your* own findings.

Interestingly, the paradigm-blasting scientist and celebrated author of *"The Hidden Messages in Water"*, Dr Emoto, maintained in his books that if you write "Love" on the microwave oven door (and on your cellphone for that matter) there are no harmful effects.[132] I find this incredible, but leave it up to you to believe it or not for yourself. Never blindly believe, or disbelieve what you are told, especially when you can validate or invalidate for yourself, but just as importantly, never dismiss anything you are told out of hand. Always ask who stands to benefit from what you are told, why, and what the possible benefits or costs to yourself and/or others to believing or accepting it may be.

A major reason that Ancient Greece could be said to have given "The Light" to the world, is that, unlike the Hebrews and Romans who were taught to "answer the question" and do what they were told, believing with "blind faith" (even if not moral), the Greeks were taught to always "question the answer" and do what is virtuous (even if not obedient), placing virtue above all else, in the quest to "Know Thyself". In fact, the enterprising and brave, disobedient person who offered alternatives was honoured and respected for the virtue of acknowledging and expressing their true selves and making a social contribution, so that, in stark contrast to the Roman and Hebrew traditions which predominate today, anyone in a symposium agreeing with anybody else was expelled from it for being spineless, lacking in imagination and not contributing anything.

This *"Hellenic Spirit"* is the heritage of all humanity and by no means the exclusive domain of those "born Greek", in the same way that the Abrahamic tradition is not the exclusive domain of Jews. You choose how to live and who you live with. Are you going to continue desperately trying to conform to a group of stuck and judgmental people for fear of being "odd" (your own unique self), or will you seek out the company of people who have the courage to be themselves and who support and approve of you as a unique individual?

Remember, that in order to expect acceptance and approval from others, you need to unconditionally accept and approve of yourself first. You then inherently command acceptance instead of begging, grovelling, hoping for it and betraying yourself. This acknowledging yourself and living your own truth and your own life is "living on purpose" and *Life* will thus support you in playing your unique role. By contrast, if you are untrue to yourself and do not play your unique role, is it not reasonable to anticipate that *Life* itself may want to "recycle" you?

5. HORMONES

"There is no one right formula for preventing breast cancer in every woman. The key to prevention of breast cancer is being aware of the various factors that cause the disease and avoiding them as much as possible, while at the same time being aware of what discourages cancerous growth in breast tissue and promoting that kind of lifestyle."
– Dr John R. Lee, M.D.[133]

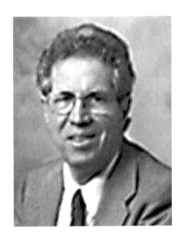

"There is no teaching force for doctors more formidable or effective than knowledgeable, intelligent, assertive women."
– Dr John R. Lee, M.D.[133]

Hormones are Awesome! They *are* the Life force! That which urges the seed to burst into life, the twig to sprout roots, the plant to flower and produce fruit; the driving force in all living beings, including you and me. And just like any driving force, in a healthy body-mind, hormones all work in harmony for optimum health and happiness, as we each travel along our own road of a meaningful Life Purpose. However, exactly because they are our powerful driving force, if they are not properly directed, balanced and not working properly; if the "driver", you and I, are overwhelmed by worry, anger or some drug or chemical, these hormones can just as easily be misdirected to cause physical and emotional (and consequently relationship) havoc at best, and at worst will cost you your life.

This myriad of health problems caused by hormonal imbalance which manifests psychologically, physically, or both, includes misdirecting our energy into the overproduction of useless or harmful cells known as cancer, according to a doctor to whom untold thousands, even posthumously, owe their lives, Dr John Lee. He was a pioneer, after Charles Huggins won a Nobel Prize in 1966 linking hormones to 8 mammalian and 7 human cancers to the 1970s,[134] into how medical 'hormones' cause cancer and how bioidentical hormones prevent, and may even reverse cancer and a host of other conditions. Dr Lee dedicated the last decade of his sadly short life (which ended in 2003) to travelling around the world at his own expense, spreading the word about hormonal imbalance and the treachery of the pseudo-hormones of the pharmaceutical industry and how people, especially women, can be empowered to regain control of their health.

His first book, which is essential reading, is *Dr Lee's Hormone Balance Made Simple*.[135] The late good Doctor wrote a number of books specifically for premenopausal *(What Your Doctor May Not Have Told You About Pre-Menopause)*[136] and postmenopausal women *(What Your Doctor May Not Have Told You About Menopause)*.[137] Both books have, to date (2016), not been disproved or superseded, but have indeed been validated by hundreds of thousands of success stories, world-wide. I would strongly recommend his books for all women, but especially women with any known gynaecological or hormonal issues, and also men over 40 *(Hormone Balance for Men*.[138]), with special reference to prostate health.

A crucial factor in a woman's hormonal life is pregnancy, which stimulates hormone production, in particular progesterone. If you are a mother and really cannot breastfeed your baby for at least two years, then feed it with a glass (not plastic) bottle and don't use other than a pure (natural, not silicone) latex teat and dummy/pacifier. I would avoid commercial "milk formula" and soy "milk" at all costs, which is invariably GM (unless explicitly stated otherwise) and in any case highly oestrogenic. There are many more alternatives to breast milk, of which the most appropriate to the child must be carefully selected, but none which substitute for the tactile and heart connection to the mother that breastfeeding provides. Then there's the vital fact that the composition of breast milk is constantly changing to give optimal nutrition to the infant as it grows. Initially it is all colostrum (cholesterol), which is vital for cell formation. Day by day, this is progressively replaced by lactic proteins, in perfect synchronization with your particular child's developmental needs. How incredibly awesome is that?

The corollary on that is that once an infant mammal matures, it loses the enzyme needed to digest the milk which renders it unsuitable, even toxic for adult consumption. In cheese fermentation milk is traditionally "pre-digested" using enzymes (rennet) from a calf's stomach,(increasingly substituted by vegetable rennet) and yoghurt is similarly "digested" using bacterial cultures, thus rendering these two dairy products digestible to adults, though the casein binding agent in cheese, particularly yellow cheeses should make the latter an infrequent part of our diet.

Pregnancies (up to two for maximum benefit; more would also in our day be ecologically irresponsible) and breastfeeding both reduce the chance of breast cancer in later life.[139] This is so for hormonal reasons, including the fact that cancer normally starts in the milk ducts which are "developed and programmed" to be used. Similarly, prostate cancer has been attributed, at least in part, to insufficient sexual activity in middle-aged men. Related to frequency of use is the psychic benefit, in both cases. Maternal nurturance is psychically linked to a woman's deep needs and life purpose – so much so that many women who do not bear children most often feel the need to either adopt a child or take on childrens' causes, as with Mother Theresa.

In no way can a sane society demean women in their role as nurturers and child-rearers. To me, moulding the future of the species is far more honourable than working for money, even though the demands of modern life often see these roles challenged and even reversed. At the end of the day, nobody should feel impelled to conform to, react against, or judge any stereotyping whatsoever.

HORMONAL ASSAULT in Modern Living

We are blissfully unaware of the preponderance of poisonous chemicals in our lives, which we inhale, eat, insert and in other ways assimilate into our bodies – to our peril. These are mostly petrochemicals, found in plastics, cosmetics, synthetic clothing, water, air pollution, food additives, packaging (especially plastic food packaging), detergents etc which unavoidably flood our everyday lives.

They enter our bodies through outgassing of petroleum derived synthetics as well as petroleum-derivative fluids, which are falsely perceived in our bodies as oestrogen, and readily taken up as such. These "false oestrogens" (or xenoestrogens (ξένο/xeno = "foreign" oestrogens), cannot be broken down or transformed into other hormones or steroids, according to its current needs for two reasons.Firstly, they are unnatural in molecular structure and the body cannot recognize or deal with them, and secondly, because even natural oestrogen is a "telic" or "end" hormone which cannot be converted, even if dangerously in excess This causes a condition of "oestrogen dominance" in both women and men.

The body needs a whole array of hormones (ορμή/orme=urge, i.e., "driving chemical"), and steroids, with the brain constantly adjusting and balancing the amount of each one in our blood and organs by means of an interactive feedback mechanism which is overwhelmed by the assault of these toxic xenoestrogens, which include pharmaceutical "hormones".

The total mind-body disruption which then occurs can manifest in an almost countless permutation of health problems, but most commonly obesity, excessive hairiness in women, head hair loss, depression, thyroid disruption, loss of libido, period problems, etc. Most notably, this is the main bodily cause of cancer, especially breast and genital cancers in both sexes.

Xenoestrogen contamination can start from conception. Although, during pregnancy, a woman is usually healthily progesterone dominant, the foetus or unborn child is still vulnerable to toxic and xenoestrogenic substances taken by the mother (whatever a mother ingests or is exposed to is experienced at a concentration five times greater by the foetus or unborn child). At infancy it is assaulted with chemicals in soaps, shampoos (especially "baby shampoos" and petroleum "baby oils"), plastic diapers and even more so the petroleum liquid-absorbing gel used with these, seriously compromising the infant's hormone system from its developmental stages.

Plastic disposable diapers also pollute the environment, taking four hundred years to decompose. Save the planet as well as your child by using eco-logical toiletries and biodegradable, interchangeable diaper inserts, or even washable diapers, as people did up to just a couple of generations ago.[140]

Women insert poisonous xenoestrogen-containing tampons deep into their bodies which, once saturated, leach chemicals readily absorbed by vaginal epithelia, together with warm waste blood which should in any case be flushed immediately from the body. The tampon and vaginal passage thus becomes an ideal breeding ground for infections, fungi and viruses. Except in "emergencies" and for brief periods of time, ladies, please use pads and even then preferably those made of non-GM cotton with non-petroleum absorbent fill. Natural, healthier and more environ-mentally responsible pads (and tampons)[141a] as well as vaginal cups[141b] are highly recommended by many women who would never revert back to commercial menstrual products.[141]

If you use a microwave oven, *never* use plastic in it, whether as a container, cover or plastic film. The container may be marked as "microwave safe", but this safety refers to the safety of the container, not to you. Why so, you ask? The microwaves, combined with plastic, will bombard your food with microscopic xenoestrogenic and carcinogenic plastic particles according to Dr Weil and an article by Dr Edward Fujimoto, PhD, Director for the Centre for Health Promotion, Castle Medical Centre, Kailua, Hawaii (mistakenly attributed to Johns Hopkins University in an article that went "viral" and can be found here).[142]

Never, ever, use chemical "air fresheners" or "deodorizers"! In fact some even have a warning on them, never to be used in closed spaces, which is where everybody uses them anyway, especially in the smallest room of the house. Don't be fooled by claims of "lavender" or "contains lemon". Unless explicitly stated otherwise, such "natural ingredients" are added in miniscule quantities just so the claim can be made. The actual active aromas and olfactory blockers are synthetic chemicals which deaden your olfactory epithelia and are highly toxic and carcinogenic.[143]

Furthermore, use even natural lavender with discretion, as this and tea tree oil are strongly phyto-(plant) oestrogenic. If you must use an "air freshener", have fun making your own, with various essential oils using an attractive clay aromatherapy burner with a beeswax candle underneath and water with a few drops of essential oil on top. Or simply use a scented beeswax candle. You may want to go more "high-tech" and use an electrical vaporizer (which works by electrically heating oil, or an oil/water mixture) or diffuser (which emits a fine spray).[144]

The same applies to deodorants. Today there are numerous natural deodorants without aluminium, sodium laurel sulphate (SLS) or any other potentially toxic chemicals, which accumulate, especially in the armpit lymphatic glands where many breast cancers start. I strongly recommend these.[145] Here again, you can have fun, exercise your creativity, save money, express your uniqueness and become less dependent making your own.[146] The same applies to detergents. Buy biodegradable, phosphate-free, unscented detergents, or make your own.[147]

If you park your car in the sun and find, upon opening the door, a strong "plasticky", xenoestrogenic smell, Dr Lee advised that you open the doors and aerate the interior to flush out the smell before entering. The same applies to the strong-smelling plastic dashboard cleaners.

How do you know whether you are oestrogen dominant, and by how much? You could get a rough idea by filling in a test quiz here,[148] or having an accurate home saliva test evaluating oestrogen & progesterone for women, or oestrogen and testosterone for men,[149] with a home testing kit or at a clinic. Ladies, please be aware that your results will be relative to the time in your menstrual cycle, so the test is best done at certain stages of your cycle with a competent health practitioner who knows the healthy range of these hormones relative to your age and stage in your cycle. Just insist on a saliva, not a blood test. Hormones are concentrated in the brain and action sites. They are not moved around in the blood constantly, but sporadically, and only when necessary. And even then, they are bound to proteins when in transit. That is why a blood hormone test is about as accurate as trying to work out the population of a city by counting all vehicles at a road checkpoint at any random time. Thus saliva, genital fluid or even urine tests are far more accurate in checking progesterone/oestrogen levels, their relative balance, as well as testosterone/androgen and oestrogen levels in men.[150]

Some medical doctors love prescribing "hormones" for just about anything. Even a young teen who is not sexually active will be put on the "pill" if she has a few pimples. Why do I write "hormones" in parenthesis? It's because pharmaceutical "hormones" are not natural human hormones, but synthetic drugs which are patented. They do share some properties in common with natural, bioidentical hormones, but also have some really nasty effects as well, as shown in the chart. Natural hormones are not patentable (so no excessive monopoly profits can be made), and thus not sold by them. One of them, Premarin® (acronym for "pregnant mare urine") is equine (horse), not human oestrogen, converted to synthetic oestrione, made from the urine of permanently penned, catheterized and immobilized, constantly artificially impregnated mares [151] until they fall over dead in their pen. Despite Premarin's® definite strong link to cancer and the unbelievably cruel conditions the mares suffer (not to mention the continuous slaughtering and discarding of foals), this drug is still widely prescribed decades after it was first introduced.

Pharmaceutical "oestrogen" is an almost guaranteed ticket to cancer, particularly breast cancer, resulting in body mutilation through breast amputation and macabre death in millions of women. So now doctors prescribe it "balanced" with "progesterone", to neutralize the cancerous oestrogenic effect. This would have been a good idea, except that the pharmaceutical substitute "progestin" is neither progesterone nor an equivalent, as fraudulently claimed by pharma companies, taught by leading universities, and believed by doctors and consequently their patients.[152]It actually worsens the situation by breaking down into oestradiol

The difference between a natural progesterone and a synthetic progestin, i.e medroxyprogesterone acetate (eg.Provera®) molecule can be clearly seen in the above diagram. Despite this, mainstream medicine cites progestin as a female hormone, as stated on the site of the prestigious Mayo Clinic on the top of my google search.[152b]

The comparison table overleaf summarises some points in Dr Lee's books.

Progestin, unlike Progesterone, breaks down into oestradiol, the most cancerous of all oestrogens, *compounding* instead of alleviating the problem of oestrogen supplementation, be it real/bioidentical oestrogen or its pharmaceutical "pirated version". Even the official US National Library of Medicine acknowledges that "balancing" oestrogen with *progestins*

NATURAL/BIOIDENTICAL PROGESTERONE	PROGESTINS (e.g. Provera ®)
Prevents Cancer	Causes Cancer
Diuretic, Reverses Bloating/Swelling	Water Retention, Bloating/Swelling
Improved Thyroid Function	----
Calming	Irritability
Anti depressant	Depressing
Maintains HDL/LDL Balance	Increases LDL ('Bad' cholesterol) Decreases HDL ('Good' cholesterol)
Stimulates Bone Regeneration (any age, even old age)	----
Increased Libido	Decreased Libido
Increased Energy	Fatigue
Improves Hair/Nails	Hair Loss
Improves Sleep	Insomnia

(synthetic "progesterone") *increases* incidence of breast cancer caused by the synthetic oestrogen, whereas the addition of natural progesterone does not.[153] To the contrary, many studies show that *natural progesterone reduces* the carcinogenic effect of the synthetic oestrogen.[154] Never, ever accept pharma "hormones". Never! If you do need progesterone, which is most likely, or oestrogen supplementation (unlikely), *always* use the natural/bioidentical plant-derived hormones, not the dangerous pharmaceutical substitutes!

Any need for oestrogen supplementation is highly unlikely, and its use strongly discouraged, as excess oestrogen, even in natural form, is highly carcinogenic, unless saliva tests at three different stages of your period, or on two occasions for menopausal women, conclusively indicate that you need it.

If your test indicates that you may be oestrogen dominant, or progesterone (women) or testosterone (men) deficient, or if you suspect it, then order *natural*, that is, *bioidentical* plant sourced progesterone cream. The best combination of optimal quality and reasonably-priced product according to my research can be ordered directly at this link.[155] As a transdermal cream, the body absorbs only what it needs, so there is no danger of an overdose, even if the recommended application of the transdermal cream is exceeded. Moreover, even if the body is "overdosed", it can be converted to whatever other hormone or steroid may be needed at the time of application, including oestrogen. Bioidentical oestrogen is also available, but unlike progesterone, oestrogen is 'telic' i.e. an "end", hormone, which if in excess, cannot be converted to anything else by the body; and we are, as mentioned already dangerously predisposed to cancer with "oestrogen dominance". It should thus only be used if *irrefutably proved* to be lacking, and not as a "treatment" for anything. Incidentally, natural/bioidentical progesterone cream, besides its unprecedented role as a cancer preventer, is the only thing that not only stops osteoporosis, but actually reverses it, without adverse effects. The world's top medical journal, the Lancet, cites a 1990 study on "the risk of breast cancer after oestrogen and oestrogen-progestin replacement" by Drs Bergkvist, Adami Ho, Persson, and others, together with Dr Lee's findings on progesterone in the reversal of osteoporosis.[156] My ex-wife, daughter, girlfriends, friends and family use and swear by natural/bioidentical progesterone. Even nutritionists emphasize the role of progesterone in breast cancer prevention, thus conceding that correct eating habits alone are not sufficient to counter the chemical assault we are subjected to in our times, and that this can only be rectified using natural progesterone cream [157]

As I am over 40, I use it to ensure excellent prostate health, (at 55 I was told that I have "an 18 year old prostate") and my hair has since stopped falling out, as it opposes DHT (dihydroxytestosterone) the major cause of hair loss in men *and* women over 35-40. I wish I had started it earlier! There are very many on the market, but at the time of writing, this progesterone cream,[158] due to its optimal concentration, consistent quality, no GMOs, price, service and all-natural ingredients in a phthalate-free container, is the one of two brands I use, praise and recommend above all. Please note that on rare occasions there may be initial (but not serious) reactions when starting on progesterone cream, (including one-off interperiod "blood spotting" in menstruating women) especially if you do not simultaneously eliminate, as far as practically possible, sources of xenoestrogens, as briefly outlined above. These issues are addressed by the excellent free support and advice through the supplier's website.

There is no justifiable reason or excuse whatsoever to take pharmaceutical pseudohormones, when these have been by far the biggest direct and indirect causes of cancer in women, especially of the breasts and reproductive organs. In Nature, synthetic hormones in women's and factory-farm animal's urine have destroyed entire riverine ecosystems, wreaking havoc even in mid-ocean, where fish species are dying out, not only due to overfishing (mainly to feed meat animals which should not be eating fish) and general pollution, but due to cancers and sexual abnormalities resulting in the inability to reproduce.[159]

Hormonal problems can, and should, be addressed with natural, bioidentical hormone creams. Because they are natural and absorbed to the extent needed, a little extra progesterone cream will not harm, unlike oestrogen. Please forgive my constant repetition that *oestrogen, even in bioidentical form, must only be supplemented when there is conclusive evidence of lack of oestrogen.* Being an "end process" hormone, unlike progesterone, it is not convertible to other hormones and steroids and is *extremely* carcinogenic when in excess. Furthermore, whilst excessive progesterone is selectively corrected by the hormonal feedback system, excess oestrogen is not. "Treating" osteoporosis with oestrogen, as is common medical practice (even if using bioidentical oestrogen), is a tragic mistake. Dr Lee points out in his books that oestrogen merely suppresses osteo*phagic* activity (the healthy dissolution of old and brittle bone to enable replacement with new bone), whilst progesterone stimulates osteo*plastic* (new bone creation) activity *at any, even old age.*[160]

I notice with alarm that products based on synthetic oestradiol (most potent and carcinogenic form of oestrogen) cream for vaginal insertion are now promoted for women with vaginal lubrication issues, without even checking for natural oestradiol levels first.[161] Not only is this (oestradiol) highly cancerous in excess, but it will contaminate her male partner, particularly if he is uncircumcised, exposing him to weight gain, gynaecomastia (breast formation or "man boobs"), and other secondary female characteristics, including cancer.

There are many other safe ways of ensuring lubrication in "dry" women which I would recommend in each particular instance, but nothing is as natural, as good and, might I say, as fun as saliva.

(If you insist on using 'medical cream' you can use bioidentical oestriol (a milder form of oestrogen) which is just as effective and does not have nearlly as strong carcinogenic effects as does excess oestradiol, however, the male partner is still exposed to this feminizing female oestrogen).

But even this is foolish, as natural progesterone cream is just as effective, and unlike the above, its "side affects" are positive for her *and* him.

More importantly, I have found that intimacy and adequate, quality foreplay has been all it takes to produce natural lubrication. Therapeutic experince has left me with no doubt that "feminine dryness" far from being the 'curse" it is made out to be, is in truth a blessing; it is the body's message, a reminder if you will, of the need and importance of (re)establishing *real intimacy*, as well as fun playfulness in all areas of our lives. Over time, we tend to become lazy and take each other for granted, whereas as we mature, the role of foreplay and intimacy should actually play a more important role. As with frigidity, it is so easy to blame the woman when the man, who generally takes the lead in sexual encounters, does not know how, or can't be bothered, to patiently and lovingly stimulate and arouse his partner. I am pleased to say that in every instance where I have done the intimacy training on couples thus far, *all* forms of apparent female and male sexual "dysfunction" have disappeared.

Regarding other uses of pharma "hormones", the ultimate birth-control benefits of the "pill" are that soon you will become either too fat for any man to be attracted to you, or you will die of cancer from the synthetic "hormones" used. Please don't do either! Should you not already be convinced, Dr Lee's books provide undisputed, *essential* reading for about-to-menstruate girls menstruating and, menopausal women, as well as men over 40 for prevention of prostatitis, prostate cancer and a healthy prostate, as bioidentical progesterone is converted to testosterone in men. It also "feeds" the testicles, whereas testosterone supplements put them "out of work" causing them to shrivel up.

The scientific hormone tracking method of contraception is considered by some to be the future of contraception.[162] It is easy, has no undesirable effects, but as a "hightech upgrade" of the traditional "timing method" may be less reliable (although its proponents offer statistics demonstrating its reliability) than most other methods, whilst avoiding the inconvenience of physical barriers and the cancer risk of IUD's and the contraceptive pill. This method may thus be more suitable for committed relationships for no barriers to intimacy or health risks.

PRACTICAL
1. Taper yourself gradually, but surely, off any synthetic hormones you may be taking, whilst simultaneously introducing natural alternatives with the support of your health care practitioner, or change to one that will cooperate with *your* life choices.
2. Do whatever is practically possible to rid yourself and your environment of xenoestrogens. Find non-toxic alternatives for commercial soaps, detergents, and disinfectants. These are just as effective and much cheaper. An excellent, must-have, all round buyer's guide is found here (it was free when I last looked but this may change).[163]
3. Don't discard your plastic dishes if you already have them, but stop using them in the microwave oven or for hot food.
4. Limit or cut out meat. Meat eaters, insist on organic meat fed on organic food naturally eaten by that species, preferably free-grazing, with no hormones or antibiotics.
5. Frequent, good sex balances hormones, tones the body, increases and balances "happy" chemicals which include serotonin, dopamine and endorphins in your body-mind. It also consumes oestradiol, which causes sexual desire, but if this desire is not expressed this hormone becomes a major carcinogen as it (in my understanding) redirects this "reproductive life force" inwards as excessive (cancerous) cell reproduction.[164]

6. THE PHYSICAL BODY

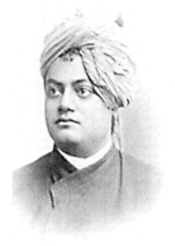

"The moment I have realized God sitting in the temple of every human body, the moment I stand in reverence before every human being and see God in him - that moment I am free from bondage, everything that binds vanishes, and I am free."
– **Swami Vivekananda** [165]

We live this life in a physical body designed to joyfully and fully participate in this world, and designed to connect physically with another. This necessitates physical wellbeing and emotional wellbeing through our personal relationship/s, which are nothing other than a yearning to find ourselves, becoming "whole," especially through a complementary other. This is a journey that, whilst expressing uniquely through each one of us as a "single note", is our contribution to the Great Symphony of Life.

It is wonderful being a top athlete, but that is not necessary. In fact, history has shown the Ancient Hellenic adage, Παν Μέτρον Άριστον/Pan Metron Ariston ("Everything in Moderation") applies here, as in all things. Extreme athletes, like those who never exercise, are nearly always outlived by the more moderate. Whilst 3, or at least 2 times a week of at least 30 minutes of disciplined exercise, not necessarily at a gym is needed, at least one exercise-session per fortnight should be out in Nature, walking, cycling, riding, surfing, etc, according to your preference, situation, age and ability.

Ensure that your exercise includes both stretching, in particular spine flexibility, and fitness/cardio-vascular work, with core work (exercising and strengthening your "core," that is your lower back to solar plexus area) and a bit of general strength training thrown in, especially for men. Yoga and Pilates are excellent for breathing and stretching, with yoga integrating spiritual components, while Pilates throws in a good core workout. It's better to do less, consistently, than to do spurts of extreme effort in the hope to "catch up" lost time which does more harm than good, confusing your metabolism.

Importantly, contrary to what you may hear, a frequent (two to three times a week, weather permitting) and moderate exposure to sunlight in the early morning and late afternoon, avoiding the "midday" sun from 11 a.m. to 2 p.m. (use your discretion depending on local conditions,) *is the best way of ensuring adequate and safe vitamin D levels, our strongest vitamin ally against cancer.* Avoid *excessive* sun. As for sun screens, do see this video[166] by Dr Coldwell before applying any. In any case, never use above factor 50 sunscreens, as their actual sunscreen effect is only marginally higher, whilst their ingredients are increasingly potentially carcinogenic. Increase internal resistance to sunburn, that is, your body's resistance to UV, by eating carotene-rich foods (natural vitamin A) such as carrots and berries. "Fortifying" sunscreens with synthetic vitamin A is no substitute for these. In fact, such "fortifying" makes them more carcinogenic than ever as the sun reacts dangerously with these chemicals, transforming them into carcinogens[166]. Aloe, avocado, coconut and olive oils offer some external protection and skin moisturizing. If you need a sunscreen, these excellent products[167] are not based on petroleum, have no carcinogens, are totally natural and highly recommended. Otherwise have fun making your own.[168] Remember that even the lightest sunscreen eliminates vitamin D production by about 93%, so soak in some rays for 10 minutes before applying any, if you feel the need to do so, more or less depending on your skin tone. Black people need longer and very pale whites need less time. Glass also blocks the solar UV frequencies responsible for vitamin D production, and due to this fact and their narrow U.V. spectrum, tanning beds paradoxically inhibit rather than facilitate vitamin D uptake! Also keep in mind that you benefit less and burn quicker by lying passively in the sun compared to moving around. You can freely access this information, video and online book with more information and invaluable advice on you and the sun.[169]

Cosmetics are an integral part of a lady's life, and also a major source of carcinogens, including aluminium, SLS, parabens and other toxic chemicals. Avoid commercial cosmetics![170]

To avoid dangerous chemicals found even in many alleged "natural" and "organic" cosmetics and skin care products, I strongly recommend these creams and cosmetics if you are in the Americas, [171] and these if you are in other parts of the world.[172] I shall keep you updated as this market develops.

THE TOUCH OF HEALTH

Massage is not an indulgence or a luxury. Ask any other mammalian mother that constantly licks her children to help them digest and ensure a good circulation in their young bodies; or a cat that keeps licking herself vigorously; or monkeys that keep "defleaing" one another; where, if there are no fleas on their companions, will put fleas on them purposely to justify the act of mutual "defleaing". In all mammals, the role of touch is essential for emotional and physical wellbeing. Animals born and raised in laboratories devoid of touch by any living being have, without exception, developed extreme psychological problems.

In the Amazon, indigenous people have a far higher survival rate with very premature babies, with the mother clutching them at her breast, than we have with incubators and technology, not to mention the "abandonment" trauma of separation from the mother and lack of touch in the latter case, which surely has lifelong consequences.

Historically, we have the central role of massage in the Ancient Greek Asklepia, and of anointing with oil and "laying of hands" in the writings of the Abrahamic religions. The importance of massage in Indian Ayurveda, Japanese Shiatzu, and other forms of body therapy throughout time and space in human history is clear. In fact, the Greek word Χριστός/Christos/Christ means "the anointed one", and having the Χρίσμα/Chrism literally means "to be anointed (rubbed down) with oil", or, in modern language, having a massage. So Jesus, in the Christian tradition, is God's way of literally physically touching, messaging/massaging, humanity as a human being.

Tragically, due to the "puritan", anti-sensual, alienating ethic of the last two millennia, the most important role of massage and touch generally has fallen into disrepute, and at the very least, massage practitioners are, in my experience, looked down upon as failures who are not capable of getting a "proper" job. The unfortunate consequence of this is that many massage practitioners have low self-esteem and consequently deliver inferior work.

We all need touch, and in particular we all need therapeutic , intentionally healing touch. This is an art-science which, other than that which to some extent may be intuitively given by a parent to a little child, has increasingly become the domain of a select few. Just as everybody needs a mechanic for their car, a plumber for their bathroom, even more so do we need a dedicated body-mind massage practitioner, not just a masseur or physiotherapist, to tend to our body-mind, ideally on a weekly basis, but at the very least once a month.

Genuine body-mind healing massage practitioners are few and far between. A genuine body-mind practitioner knows that theory and technique, whilst important, is secondary to total dedication and real heart-centred connection with the recipient. There is a world of difference between receiving a massage from such a person and just feeling a "pair of hands of your average salon masseuse going through the motions" on you.

Furthermore, such a person, though confident, is humble, as s/he knows that true healing is not something they *do, but a process they facilitate,* and allow to happen *through* them, and with a deep Heart connection and the consent and cooperation of the client. The greatest challenge for such a healing practitioner is to respect a client's choice to stay in denial and remain 'closed' to a greater or lesser extent,.or to progress at the rate with which the latter is comfortable. Healing, unlike therapy cannot be imposed. It is a choice, and the choices and the relationship between the treated and the healer must be clearly defined with the cooperative, respectful leadership of the healer.

Why do we need massage, and especially a body-mind healing massage? Anybody that has ever had a good massage given by a dedicated body-mind healer, or even a good "regular" masseur knows the answer to that. It is an answer that, like everything else that *really* counts in Life, cannot be satisfactorily expressed by the limitations imposed by words, let alone measures.

The benefits of massage looked at in a purely reductionistic, physical and "left-brained" way are that it relaxes muscles and the body, and also stimulates blood circulation and lymph drainage. However, it is far more than this; firstly, we need massage to restore physical and emotional balance. We also need it to enable us to leave the prison of the head and enter (back into) the Heart, and to open up the energy pathways of which the ancient Chinese, Hellenes, and Indians knew thousands of years ago, and which our science is only recently and begrudgingly beginning to understand and acknowledge.

Additionally, and most relevantly, the tragically dismissed fact is that a therapeutic massage given by a skilled healer uncovers deep emotional/physical blocks, most of which we have long since suppressed and forgotten, but which remain in our body-mind, slowly, but ever-so surely, silently poisoning us.

The pharma/medical approach is to keep suppressing the expression of such issues. The healer's function is to work with you to identify, accept, embrace and transcend such emotional and physical issues so that they are resolved early, before they escalate into debilitating illness and even death, instead of,as we have been conditioned, to deny our physical (and emotional) symptoms, through pharmaceuticals, until it's too late.

That is why the wise avoid the sorcerer's (pharmaceutical) path, but rather seek out the assistance and guidance of a body-mind healer to seek out such disharmonies, becoming aware of them earlier rather than later. Then, by the blocks and subtle sensations, pain and "symptoms", the underlying "messages" are dis-covered and such wise and self empowered people undertake to process them psycho-emotionally, with the therapist/healer who simultaneously manually works on releasing our physical blockages

The similarity of the words "massage" and "message" is most

certainly not "mere coincidence", but enshrines a far deeper meaning; of conveying a "message" of self-awareness that words alone can never impart

For those who appear to be less fortunate, who do not have regular therapeutic body-mind or even "regular" massage therapy, or whose state of denial is more vigorous, there may not be such minor warning signs, or they may be suppressed, intentionally or unintentionally, as our emotional war against ourselves turns into full-scale physical war which could take the form of a heart attack, a stroke, or cancer. A good body-mind healer, always with our cooperation, will uncover emotional and physical blocks *before* they become a major issue, which is why, especially after a first session you may even feel unwell. This is known as a "healing crisis," or in the case of (the release of) physical toxins, the so-called "Herxheimer Effect", a transitional phase which must be understood as such.

In a deeper sense, all dis-ease is, in fact, a "healing crisis" which, if resisted,only becomes more intense, and eventually leads to premature death. But if accepted, acknowledged and acted on and *truly healed or transcended*, the crisis, by definition, takes you, *not* to a point you were before the symptoms which the crisis manifested, but to a far higher level of body-mind "wellbeing" than before the state which preceded it, and which in actual fact, (unbeknown to you) created the diagnosed condition.
It is *precisely your body-mind state before* (often many years before) a dis-ease (including cancer), *that caused the physical manifestation of the disease in the first place*. Directly or indirectly.

So it bears repeating once again, that it is not the "symptom" or "crisis" that needs healing, *but the body-mind state which led up to it*. It is like the motor "accident": Panel-beating, or body-shop work, may make a temporary cosmetic change, but does not solve the problem. In fact it masks it. Unlearning your "bad driving habits" first, *then* learning to "drive better", *does* solve your "accident" problem before you have another "collision", which could cost you your life.

The relationship between your body-mind healer and yourself

is a unique, privileged and sacred one.

The quality of this relationship, this connection, is more important than the modality of treatment itself, this being the means through which the healing is communicated.

In my experience in this life-long committment, I have long since let go of epithets such as "psychology", "counselling", "aromatherapy", "massage", "shiatsu", "reflexology", "Reiki", "EFT", "NLP", "Swedish massage" etc., as these are merely therapeutic moulds in which a learner-healer can start, before outgrowing and transcending them. The mature healer is not just a therapist, a psychologist,doctor, reflexologist, energy therapist or "an" anything. A real healer is not replicable, let alone certifiable or franchisable. A healer, whilst learned and knowledgeable, is *essentially* Him/Her Self. Nothing more, certainly nothing less. It is all about integrating knowledge, intuition, and heart connection in the here and now, not imposing, but guiding the recipient from creating dis-ease due to ignorance and fear, to health through self-enlightenment, taking us back to the timeless *Delphic Maxim*, "Know Thyself".

For those again who are extremely "left-brained," generally (but not always), men, for whom the "full picture" is too broad, intangible, too "hazy" or "too much," and who prefer to analyse, let's look at some specific benefits of the integrated body-mind approach.

As mentioned, physical precursors of cancer include poor oxygen supply and acidity. A vigorous massage stimulates blood circulation (and thus supply and availability of fresh oxygenated blood) and breaks down blockages, improving oxygenation, and assists in detoxing by getting lymph (which has no vascular system) moving, and cleansing the body of acidity, in particular uric and lactic acids, secreted by muscles, especially by people who exercise. So, people who exercise do not need massage any less, but generally for relatively different physical benefits. Indeed, most of my clients have been physically fit younger women, which presently tends to be the most psycho-physically aware sector of the population.

One instance where massage is directly related to the prevention of cancer is breast cancer, either by a skilled therapist, healer, or partner, or taught to, and administered by, the woman herself, at least once a week. It must not be undertaken as an act of anxiety, but as an act of love. Do not underestimate the power of the mind (in the broader, not merely cerebral sense) combined with touch! Breast cancer may start in the milk ducts or be caused by the accumulation of toxins stuck in the lymph glands/nodes, (which are intended to *clear* such toxins) and as such may start in the armpits, which makes it especially important to not use chemical deodorants which are readily absorbed here, and *never even think about using antiperspirants*.[173] The skin is our biggest excretory organ. Indeed, if our entire skin surface was to be stopped from breathing and excreting, we would almost instantly die. To prevent perspiration entirely would be akin to and as deadly as plugging up your anus!

If you need a deodorant, there are natural deodorants on the market such as these.[174] Alternatively, you can make one yourself, or even use colloidal silver, or plain or naturally perfumed sodium bicarbonate paste, to control the bacteria in sweat which cause the disagreeable odour when they die off. (unless you have candida or another health issue, a healthy body does not of itself have a disagreeable odour) Unlike commercial deodorants, these will not poison you or destroy your all-important pheromones[175].

Keeping "a-breast" of our present issue, studies have shown that no less than 85% of women wear ill-fitting bra's, causing constriction of lymph drainage directly linked to cancer, especially with underwire bra's.[176] Synthetic fabric bra's cause heating of the breast and prevent normal "breathing" (of the skin), another contributer to cancer, hence the banning of synthetic bras in Russia in October 2014. Remember, women have done very well "hanging free" without loss of firmness, until bra's were invented just over 100 years ago as a fashion statement, and studies have shown that, all things being equal, women not wearing bras are less likely to come down with breast cancer.[177] Furthermore, breast sagging has nothing to do with not wearing a bra. In fact, recent studies have proved quite the opposite![177d]

The best thing to do if you want firm, healthy breasts is to keep fit, not smoke, and not put on weight and then lose it (especially if done so quickly or in feast-famine spurts) and (the part you will enjoy most), massage them![177e] The subject of breast cancer merits its own book. Contact me if interested in a free preview of a book breast cancer; in addition to Dr Lee's book: *What your Doctor May Not Tell You About Breast Cancer.*[178]

Another form of massage specifically aimed at preventing cancer is prostate massage. Prostate cancer is the most common cancer in men, often following the all too common non-malignant problem of prostatitis. As men get older, the prostate tends to enlarge, and as the sex drive drops, the seminal vesicles clog up just as with the lobules, or milk glands, in women's breasts. Prostate massage keeps the prostate "healthy" and "milking the prostate" by a skilled prostate masseuse clears congested seminal vesicles.[179] Alternatively, one can buy a prostate massage "wand" specifically designed for the purpose.[180] Sexual arousal elicited by prostate massage is natural in heterosexual as well as homosexual males and is not an indicator of sexual orientation. Prostate massage will certainly improve and maintain your sexual performance, as well as stave off incontinence, as do "Kegel" exercises which stimulate blood flow and condition the muscles of the pelvic basin, general pelvic health and improve sexual performance in men and women.[181] Prostate protection and treatment is also dealt with in Dr Lee's book: *Hormone Balance For Men.*[182] You won't hear any of Dr Lee's life-saving advice for men and women from your average doctor.

SEXUALITY

Our perverted sense of imposed "morality" has denied us the realisation that the sexual part of our physicality is the link between our physical, emotional, social and even (especially?) spiritual selves, and imbalances here have been the cause of many a cancer, so making mention of this vital issue essential. In this respect, "seven chakra massage" – in other words, massage of the entire body, including sexual release of men and women , has its place when done with established clients by request. I have also trained numerous couples in the art of "Seven Chakra Massage", taking them methodically from head to toe. This is the greatest investment a couple can ever make in itself. All couples so far who have done the workshop have asserted that it has taken their relationship holistically to heights that they could never have imagined, even in their wildest spiritual, romantic or hedonistic dreams. Contact me to make the best of your time together. There is no second chance to make the most of your vitality, your relationship and your life, and every day lost is lost forever, and leaves you with a day less .[183]

Sexual attraction and bonding is an expression of Eros, the Universal Principle of Attraction, Creation, Procreation and Completion. The whole Universe and everything in it, runs on it. In humans, it is symbolically acted out through our sexuality. The extent to which we relate healthily with our own erotic expression, as expressed through sexuality is to a large degree reflected in our lives as a whole. So how you express your sexuality has everything to do with you, and you cannot understand, accept or love yourself (and by projection, anybody else) unless you accept and love this central aspect of yourself, unconditionally.

Society has imprisoned us with rules based on superstition, fear, guilt, "shoulds" and "should nots", "rights" and "wrongs", which are not only unrelated to love and acceptance or reason, but arise from the exact opposite: judgment based on unquestioned and even fanatically promoted social, religious and other authoritarian doctrines. So, in most of us, to a greater or lesser extent, the divine Erotic force, instead of bringing us wholeness, causes us inner conflict and guilt, perverting our relationship with ourselves and by projection, the complementary sex. Sexual perversion or obsession never arises from its spontaneous loving expression in whatever form, but to the contrary, by its demonization, suppression and denial.

This applies all the more so to sexual minorities. Whereas, for instance, most people seek physical and emotional completion in the complementary sex, some people feel complemented/complete with, and are thus attracted to, the same sex. Whether it is because they are "female souls trapped in a male body" or vice-versa, or genetic or environmentally determined, that is the way it is. It is nothing to be ashamed or proud of (Such "pride" is actually reactive or a denial of shame). Moreover, it is nobody else's business; small is the mind that fixates on anything, including sexuality, especially when it concerns someone else.

As mentioned in the obviously connected chapter on hormones, cancer is particularly linked to a predominance/surplus of oestrogen, especially its most potent form, oestradiol, which also tends to be disproportionately overrepresented in pharma "oestrogens". Oestradiol, amongst other functions, (like progesterone) is involved with sex drive. There are generally two reasons for excess oestradiol in particular (other than pharma "hormones"). The one is xenoestrogens (from petrochemicals) which tend to be oestradiol dominant and the other is that the oestradiol is not allowed to be used up doing its job of getting you to express yourself sufficiently sexually, qualitatively as well as quantitatively.

Some, actually most, people have secret fetishes, preferences and sexual fantasies (so you see! It's not just you! ;-) which, though they could (and "should") be expressed between mutually benefitting adults, seldom if ever are. Or if they are, may elicit great guilt, as these are frowned upon by religion, parents (who most likely had their own fetishes which they were too afraid to express) and a hypocritical society.

A sex drive that is not acted upon and fulfilled (which means to be expressed in the way that is truly *you*, not the way that society or doctrines dictate) is a first class ticket to cancer, particularly genital cancers. This essential part of our lives has fallen victim to a cancerous lifestyle of "all work and no play", and even when there is "play", it is all too often out of a sense of duty. If you don't have a partner, while it is by no means the same, utilize "self-service" as a stop-gap, though not a replacement.

On the other hand, here, as everywhere, take everything in moderation. Excessive emphasis/fixation on sexuality is not a spontaneous self-expression but one of desperation and addiction.

Another interesting phenomenon on the increase, as relationships are becoming increasingly heart (centre/chakra)-based, and less genitally based (the lower two psychophysical centres/chakras are about physicality, possessiveness and ownership), is an increasing number of people who do not consider sex as the unique expression of connection between them. Thus, there are increasing instances both of "no sex marriages" and "open marriages". No type of relationship is "right" or "wrong" and no adult couple is answerable to anyone else or any social or other "belief" system. In fact no intimate partnerhip may be in true integrity if it subordinates itself to social, family and other expectations True partnership is based on mutual agreement, integrity and respect of one's own true nature and that of the other. Quite clearly then each relationship lived in integrity has the potential of being unique and special far beyond any of the fairy-tale imposed "one-size-fits-all" expectations on which we have been raised and indoctrinated to believe.

The bottom line is, that in whatever form it takes, you need to honour yourself enough to allow you to express yourself, including sexually when those feelings arise within you, provided that this comes from a space of joy and not of neediness, anger or deceit; or to please, possess, control, win-over, avenge etc. A woman who feels so lowly of herself that she needs to use sex as an escape or to buy favour will have her own negative judgement reflected back to her by cruel, judgmental (i.e. hypocritical) people in a society which condemns sexual excess in women and commends it in men. This is thanks to a hypocritical religious tradition which makes sexual gratification the prerogative of men while simultaneously making it the shame of the "sinful" woman.

This acceptance of self, of course, does not apply to imposing your will on the weak, such as in paedophilia or violent sexual assault. If you feel that way inclined, acknowledge it (don't try to deny it, or judge yourself, as this will only exacerbate it), and *seek help before acting it out*. This inclination demonstrates that you feel inadequate to deal with an adult and/or that you have much anger which was not expressed adequately and appropriately and is now expressing itself in a cowardly way at helpless victims. Many paedopphiles reenact having been so abused themselves Conversely, those that like being beaten up themselves were probably beaten a lot by a parent and unconsciously associate violence with what they have been taught to believe is love.

When we "fall into a hole", figuratively as well as physically, we need somebody "outside" to drop us a lifeline. We cannot do it alone, just as we cannot expect another to climb out on our behalf. (Like the drowning man who prayed to God to be saved, refusing all human assistance; who, as anecdote goes, after drowning was in the afterlife reprimanded by God who had sent all the people to save him.) Having counselled and helped such people, I can honestly say that everybody so afflicted, with the correct counselling, *without exception*, found that an affectionate and mutually rewarding relationship with another adult is both possible and far more satisfactory and fulfilling, both immediately and long term. And the vicious cycle of guilt, anger and fear of persecution leading to more such violent and exploitative acts is over, permanently, to be replaced with a healthy "virtuous cycle" of increasing love, integration and self-acceptance.

Just as importantly, such people that I have counselled at some stage eventually acknowledged that the violence expressed outwards was no more than the expression of "a cancer eating themselves from within". Indeed, victims of such people are a "metastasis" of this "cancer", whether or not it becomes physically manifested. The famous "affirmations" writer, Louise Hay, has written how she manifested uterine cancer from being raped as a child, and how she healed what the doctors said was a terminal condition by acknowledging, forgiving, and transcending it. I recommend some books of hers, in particular this one.[184] For those who have the courage and integrity to acknowledge, and the determination to transcend paedophilia, either as tendency, fantasy, perpetrator or victim and choose me as your counsellor, you will by no means be the first or the last I will have successfully assisted.

Even without being exposed to the overt sexual violence of rape and paedophilia, the healthy expression of your sexuality may be extremely difficult in certain situations, including not feeling emotionally and/or sexually fulfilled with your partner, in which case you are, in reality, not being faithful to your partner. How can you be, if you are not even faithful to yourself? Do you not owe it to *yourself* to be fulfilled, emotionally and physically, and does your partner not deserve to have someone who can give of her/himself fully and with no reservation? Would you like someone to be with you out of a "sense of duty", possibly even imagining another person, or in other fantasy scenarios, while physically engaged with you?

You only live once. Whether your soul reincarnates or not is irrelevant. So live genuinely, honestly, and lovingly. It's not always easy, but emotional denial and turbulence will cause you unnecessary suffering, and sooner or later manifest pathologically in some way in your body. So, hard as it may be, being true to yourself is infinitely better than the alternative, for you and for anyone with whom you are relating. Remember, *integrity* is the act of *integrating* all parts of *yourself*, first and foremost The moment you deny part/s of yourself, (whether physical, intellectual, emotional or spiritual parts) those parts will protest and your health (not to mention relationships) will suffer, first in your mind, then your actions, to finally manifest in physical disease.

PRACTICAL
1. Physical Exercise. Are you on a disciplined exercise program thrice, or at least twice a week? If not, commit to it now. Your exercise must include flexibility, stamina and strength training (more of the latter for men) in that order, according to your age and condition. The trick is not to set an all-time achievement record immediately, but to do even a little, consistently. Take out your diary, and make a commitment – now. It is easier if you can commit to set classes, but if your budget does not allow for it, you will have to make up the difference with disciplined commitment.
2. Sexual Expression. Are you sexually frustrated? Sexual connection starts with communication. If you are not communicating satisfactorily with your partner, take responsibility and do something about it, but failing in a *genuine* attempt to do so, move on. If you are unattached, single, get out there and meet people, lots of people, and have fun meeting various people, especially with groups that share your interests. Do it unconditionally and without any expectations, or you will just be perceived as a "creep". Be yourself, and trust nature to find a way. It's that simple.
3. Find a body-mind practitioner, at least an "ordinary" masseur/masseuse, one who is non-judgemental,

with whom you can let go completely, and trust with confidentiality. Go for weekly sessions, or at least once a month, and negotiate a regular patronage discount in return for paying monthly upfront, as I do with my clients.

7. ACIDITY AND FUNGUS

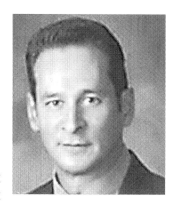

"Cancer is a fungus"
– **Dr. Tullio Simoncini, Italian oncologist, famous for curing "incurable" cancers with cheap ingredients from your kitchen cupboard. See a video on him.**[185]

Dr Simoncini's assertion that "cancer is a fungus" does not contradict Warberg's hypothesis that cancer comes from oxygen deprivation, but supports it, as acidity and oxygen deprivation are two aspects of the same thing and, as such, are themselves the necessary conditions for fungal infection.

The three immediate precursors of cancer are:
1. – oxygen deprivation, leading to...
2. – an acid system *(or vice versa.)*... which invariably leads to the breakdown of acids to sugars, which ferment through...
3. – anaerobic or partially anaerobic fungal infection, in most cases Candida albicans, but also other fungi and viruses (eg HPV- though this is now disputed)

That fungus is *the* precursor to cancer is supported by many cures of "incurable cancers", simply by eliminating associated fungal infection. Introduced by Italian Dr Simoncini, and backed by leading authorities throughout the world, including the Mayo Clinic and Johns Hopkins University in the U.S., elimination of fungal infections through administration of alkaline, antifungal bicarbonate of soda (aka baking soda), straight out of your kitchen cupboard) saved the breasts and lives of many women. (Repeat: Baking soda is not to be confused with

Baking Powder® which contains other chemicals including toxic aluminium).

In a possible forthcoming book on the natural, affordable, painless and effective transcendence of cancer, various simple but most efficient methods, including ways of administering sodium bicarbonate, are amongst the proven modalities discussed. If you are interested in the book, or a skype consultation now, please contact me.[186]

Although it is quite natural to have a small presence of *Candida albicans* in the gut, in an increasing number of people, the Candida population far exceeds the tolerable size and is out of control, escaping first through a weak ileocecal valve from the large intestine(where it is needed) to the small intestine (where it becomes pathological) and then the confines of the gut to penetrate deep into body tissues and organs.

Most obvious possible symptoms include genital or anal itching in both sexes, but Candida can run rampant in just about any part of the body, even the brain, and thus, just like hormonal imbalance, can result in almost any seemingly unrelated symptoms, physical and psychological. In the gastro-intestinal tract it consumes nutrients in your food like a tapeworm, before you can digest and assimilate them. Its secretions are poisonous and further increase the acidity in your system which, in turn, makes the environment more favourable for itself and for the formation of cancer cells. Furthermore, candida 'hijacks' your appetite, causing you to crave the sugar and refined carbohydrates on which it thrives.

Not everyone with Candida, genital warts or other fungi will be struck by cancer, but cancers, according to Dr Simoncini's findings, start with the white fungal infection: Candida *albicans*. (*alba=white,Lat.*) So, why not simply eliminate yourself from the cancer risk list by freeing yourself of Candida?

Firstly, how do you know whether you are a Candida sufferer? If you keep scratching down under, have oral or vaginal thrush or cystitis, or itch anywhere in your body, suffer from depression, lethargy or confusion, or even bad breath or body odour, Candida may well be the cause.

There are various tests for Candida: **Firstly**, laboratory tests, at a clinic or at home, which tests for three Candida antibodies[187], and which are expensive and unreliable. **Secondly,** more subjective quiz tests, such as this one,[188], and **Thirdly,** a quick, simple and an old favourite, conducted as follows:

Before sleeping at night, put a glass of unchlorinated water at your bedside. (If you only have tap water, boil it initially to vaporize the chlorine). First thing upon rising the following morning, spit into it. Look at it approximately every 15 minutes for up to 45 minutes. If you do not have a throat infection and there are "strands" descending downwards from your floating spittle, that is a sure sign of Candida. Though seemingly simplistic, I've learnt to trust this method way above expensive lab tests which can only make inferences from antibodies and so in my opinion inaccurate.

If you seek 'expert diagnosis,' you will find no consensus; generally medical diagnosticians are biased towards a negative and non medical therapists towards a positive identification of the fungus, which is considered to be the most underdiagnosed disease of our times.

With such a serious parasite and indeed cancer precursor, I would always recommend erring on the side of caution. Rest assured that the treatment protocols suggested here have no undesirable , but only positive ("side") effects, whether or not you have a Candida issue. Indeed many people such as I take them every two years. Prevention is always better and infinitely wiser than cure.

Candida infestation can be due to junk food, especially sugar and white bread, carbonated/fizzy drinks, being emotionally compromised and/or stressed (as mentioned in the section on emotions), live in a chemically, emotionally and electromagnetically polluted environment, or, most likely, all of the above.527 Anyone untouched by any of the above, and not on your own Pacific island, please raise your hand.

It is much easier cultivating a habit of healthy eating than having to do a three months fast excluding *everything* but non starch vegetables nuts, seeds and healthy plant oils. If you think you may possibly have Candida, take action immediately! At best it could save your life and, at worst, it won't hurt you. There are no adverse (so-called "side-") effects, to either protocol, which can only benefit you and will minimize your chances of falling prey to the fungus for at least a year of healthy living thereafter.

The traditional intervention for Candida, which takes a long time and a great deal of discipline for success, includes a good probiotic such as acidophilus and the brand I recommend is this one.[189] But for quicker, easier and more effective treatment you may prefer[190], being the increasingly preferred way for quick and with guaranteed results. Your life is far too valuable to take *any* chances at all! Both options are 100% safe and many people, including myself, use these prophylactically (preventatively), although for prophylactic reasons the first acidophilus treatment, *if* you have the inclination or discipline to eat *uncompromisingly* healthily should be sufficient . Are you keen to make your own probiotics, for free?Then do it![190b,c]

Regardless as to whether you have any symptoms of Candida, I still recommend that you maintain a healthy diet with at least 70% vegetables and a few fruits *between, not after* meals, as outlined in the "Foods" section – and no processed sugar (or foods containing it), this being the primary food of fungi and cancer cells, not to mention the cause of type 2 diabetes. Use honey sparingly (it is greatly beneficial in moderation, i.e under a tablespoonful a day for most of us) or buy concentrated stevia fluid. Liquid stevia is generally purer than powdered stevia, has no bitter aftertaste and, unlike the solid stevia, is more accurately measurable and evenly distributed in a drink or bake mix alike. Stevia is safe and much sweeter than sugar, so miniscule amounts are needed, and it's reputedly even beneficial for diabetics and people with cancer. Even better, if you have warm weather and a sunny spot, grow your own stevia plant and use the pulverized dried leaves! However, be warned! What you have *not been told* is that Stevia has been traditionally used by indigenous people in Paraguay and central America by women as a most effective fertility inhibiter, so *dont use it if you intend falling pregnant!!* (Its effectiveness lasting two months after you stop taking it). On the other hand, I am not endorsing it as a foolproof contraceptive either.

As mentioned, even if you do not appear to have a Candida problem, what I do, and thus highly recommend, is take an acidophilus[189] course in any case if you have (*much*) more discipline than money; or this one,[190] if you have less discipline than money, or if your life is already too complicated, like most of us. Repeat it at least every two years in the summer (when you eat less). Both are natural, and can only do you good. Definitely *always* take a course of acidophilus if you are on antibiotics, or even make your own probiotics which are at least as good as shop bought probiotics.[189cd] Eating yoghurt (without gelatin and other additives) is good, but not enough when on antibiotics; and acidophilus has proven to be the probiotic of choice. Greek yoghurt has the well-earned reputation of being the best in the world and is further thickened to a quarter of its volume by straining. However, in other countries, "Greek" yoghurt is usually plain yoghurt artificially thickened (instead of strained) for profit maximization and is to be avoided, having none of the benefits of Greek yoghurt but all of the hazards of synthetic chemicals. Plain yoghurt, with no added or subtracted fat is best, and sheep or goat yoghurt if you can get it is far healthier than that of cow's milk, especially commercial pasteurized cow's milk. Finally, ensure from the label that the yoghurt *contains* live cultures, not simply *made with* live cultures.[191]

PRACTICAL
1. Put a glass of water at your bedside now, so that you can test yourself tomorrow, as you rise.
2. If you have any symptoms of possible Candida infection, you may confirm this with a quiz or clinical lab test and treat it immediately! Remember; Better safe than sorry!
3. If on antibiotics, *definitely* take a course of acidophilus,[189] preferably whilst still on them or as soon as possible thereafter. This is *not* an option. Yoghurt is a helpful dietary probiotic, but not enough to counter antibiotics.

8. MEDICINE & ANTIBIOTICS

"You may have thought cancer or heart disease takes the lives of more Americans than any other illness or event. But conventional medicine is actually the leading cause of death today!"
– **Dr. Josh Axe**[192]
Also see *"Death by Medicine"* by five Medical Doctors, two with PhDs [193]

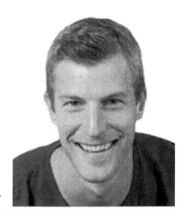

"The medical curriculum was created by John D Rockefeller over 100 years ago when he produced chemicals and didn't know how to sell those chemicals. He produced sales people and called them MDs. He produced the entire curriculum for the education of medical doctors. Rockefeller made sure that the medical doctor never learned how to cure. A medical doctor has about 1 hour of education in diet and nutritional health and no knowledge of healing. They study pathology which is the study of decay and death. They study the chemical intervention of symptoms; they don't study healing, curing or looking for the root cause of disease. The only cause for any kind of disease is the lack of energy and that's mainly caused by physical or emotional stress."[194]
– **Dr Leonard Coldwell**

(It thus follows that...)
"The medical doctor statistically has the shortest lifespan of 56 years, the highest abuse ratio of alcohol and drugs, the highest suicide rate (only psychiatrists have higher) and you go to...(them)...to ask them how to have a happy, long life."[194b]
– **Dr. Leonard Coldwell**

Very few of us realise the role of "medicines" in creating the ideal conditions for cancer in our body. This is because people have been indoctrinated (in-*doct*-rinated) into unquestionably believing that the purpose of the pharmaceutical industry, and the related genetic "modification" industry, is to heal and feed, respectively. However, even with the simplest logic, we can see that these are dangerously false and misleading assumptions, considering these industries' ethics, "value" systems, and track record as developers and manufacturers of toxic chemicals, and especially their intended use against humanity and our living environment.

Quite apart from that, what is the purpose of a business, in pure capitalistic terms? Profit maximization, right? So if you own a restaurant you want hungry people, if you sell champagne you want celebrators, if you are an undertaker or mortician you profit greatly when a busload of school children drives off a cliff. A tow truck driver in my hometown wanted to create business and was arrested for pouring oil on the road for cars to skid on. Extreme, but tragically true and relevant. Likewise, Anton Rupert, the South African tobacco billionaire, having created a flourishing lung cancer market, moved into the "after sales service" of hospitals. (I am not suggesting that it was his intention in the first instance, while on the other hand I also doubt that he was unaware of the relationship of smoking to lung cancer, and neither do I know whether he smoked or not).

The purpose of the pharmaceutical industry, just like any other business, is to maximize profits, and it does so by ensuring that people are sick and (paradoxically) dependent on them, with the support of the media and governments, both of which they effectively own.

So is the cancer industry a success? Well, have they succeeded in the cardinal rules of:

1. Creating a market?
   Possibly, through poisoning, let's read on and see.
2. Cornering the market?
   Yes, with media promotion,your unquestioning support, government legislation and ruthless suppression of alternatives.
3. In keeping/retaining customers?

Yes! Their "therapeutic techniques" for chronic diseases including diabetes, cancer, MS, etc keep people (barely) alive for as long as possible before a most gruesome death. (In chemo, tumours almost always shrink initially, giving false hope).

It bears repeating that the cancer industry is an overwhelming success, and (tragically) a prime example of what constitutes a top world class business, an "inspiration" for all hardnosed "bottom liners" and a sure bet for your investment (unless of course you die of cancer before your shares rise sufficiently). Woe betide anyone who should threaten this massive monopolistic industry with a cure! Google "alternative doctors killed"! This is what happens when we sacrifice human values for profits; we create a monster which turns back and consumes us!

But, just a minute, isn't this a definition of cancer? So the world is trusting a worldwide predatory and cancerous organization to treat....cancer!?

Let's put things into perspective.
Just like a troubled (perceived and judged as "naughty") child, an unhealthy body needs to be understood regarding how and why it relates to its environment the way it does, and supported rather than punished with toxic chemicals like chemo, life killing (anti-biotic) potions for infections (a safe alternative is offered in our book), and dangerous, mind-distorting drugs for people who don't conform to the mass-minded idea of reality. Such "treatments and cures" exacerbate existing problems and/or create new problems, if not immediately, then at some point down the line. The effect is thus to create more business, hooking you into a lifelong downward spiral. As with the "naughty" child, we need to notice the symptom and respond with compassionate understanding to identify and treat the root cause. This is how we take response-ability for our lives instead of resisting the results of our thoughts and actions which life presents us, and continuing to give away this right, power and responsibility to individuals and interest groups who further their own agenda, at our expense.

Look how far we have allowed ourselves to be grossly misled in our relationship to Life.

Germs or "microbes" (μικρό/micro=small, βίο/bio=life) are literally "small life forms". You need a microscope to see them. Neither good, nor bad, these small life forms are essential for the existence and survival of "macrobes",(μακρό/macro=large) that is, large life forms, or organisms, such as you, me, your cat, and the cockroach. Without micro-organisms (microbes) in your stomach to enable you to digest and assimilate your food, you would die of starvation. Without microbes in the soil, we would have no plants, and no life as we know it on the planet at all.

Yet it is these selfsame microbes essential for the creation of food, as well as for its digestion, and life itself, that we lump with many other micro-organisms which we blame for illness, for we have been indoctrinated to fearfully go on an all-out rampage; to kill and destroy all microbes, (i.e. life itself!) as with anything we can't see or understand, big or small.

Let's look at *e-coli* for instance, the very mention of which causes extreme panic. Its home is in our large intestine, (along with the Candida fungus) performing an essential task in our digestion, keeping us alive. Now surely we should be full of gratitude to such a self-demeaning fellow. Would *you* dedicate *your* life to living up someone's backside in order to keep them alive and healthy? Hmmm…. Maybe I should retract that statement, as so many of us fearfully live that way, "creeping up other people's asses" and then resenting ourselves……and we all know what chronic resentment causes.

The problem lies not with the microbe, but with our *relationship* with the microbe. Who told us to deposit the *e-coli* bacterium in what used to be pristine waters? Is it not then divine justice that the selfsame water should, in turn, poison us? There are many ways to look at this dynamic: In religion it is known as "reaping what you sow", "karma", "kismet", "God's will", etc; in biology it is referred to as a self-regulating system, where the water ecology, in order to survive, must eliminate its poisoner; in physics it is referred to as Newton's Second Law; and in Systems Theory, a Closed Loop.

E-coli also comes from animal products, when they are raised, slaughtered and "processed" in certain inhumane ways. You may object, saying that this is not the only microbe, and that there are other "baddies". Nature is a system designed to manifest Life by sustaining, improving and evolving itself (not necessarily in the Darwinian sense). As such, She uses Her resources economically. If She sees any living form that is not fulfilling its purpose, that is weak and not purposeful in its mission, whatever it may be, She will claim back its body for recycling into something else. But when we are sick, and the doctor, quite oblivious to the Big Picture, diagnoses (or rather the laboratory identifies) a certain bacterium or "bug," it is immediately villainized and we bomb ourselves with antilife (mainly fungal) preparations and chemicals, which we call antibiotics (anti-life/living in Greek).

What we should rather be doing is desisting from confusing the messenger with the cause, and poisoning it and ourselves. We should stop answering bad questions, and instead question the answers which we have for so long blindly accepted. Why has Life presented me with this influenza (in this case a virus, unresponsive to antibiotics anyway) which will cause me to rest for a week? Is it because I overwork? Do I need a rest? Is it a "safety valve" for me? Is it because I am working at (what for me and my Life Purpose is) the wrong thing? And that I need to reassess/meditate/pray over, or reconsider it?

If I have a headache, do I resist it and take a pill to mask the pain? We have all heard of the person "of perfectly good health" who just suddenly fell dead with a stroke for "no rhyme or reason" when, unbeknown to anyone, he kept on ignoring gentle warnings by wiping them out with a "headache pill"…

When-your-car-makes a grinding noise, do you merely turn up the radio? When the red light flashes on the dashboard, do you simply remove the 'guilty' bulb, or break it with a hammer?

We presently live in a "world culture" of unconsciousness, denial, and meaninglessness. Instead of having an economic system to serve us, we are slaves to it. Every dollar you "make" is in reality an I.O.U that just adds to overall worldwide debt. We perpetuate fear by electing people and lifestyles that exploit and magnify those fears. Whether it be a politician (i.e. a cell in a cancerous political system), a carcinogenic deodorant, or another "must-have gizmo" which will, before we know it, be thrown onto the never-ending pile of toxic waste, just to be replaced with a "newer and better" version.

We are living lives of addiction – addicted to "stuff" (materialism), to people (addictive/possessive relationships, hero worship), beLIEfs (political, religious, scientific, philosophical etc), *junk* food, sugar, coffee, porn, drama, chocolate, money. These, and countless other forms of addiction, cause us to distract, demean, disempower and destroy ourselves as we give our power to things of infinitely less value than ourselves, other people, the ecosystem (οίκος/ecos=home) and our Life Mission, whatever it may be.

All that "modern medicine" has achieved is to kill the messenger and burn the message, changing the way we live, suffer and die. When the mind and spirit object, psychiatric drugs or "medicines" are used to bring us "back into line". When the body protests, medicines are used to "fight the illness". We are so addicted to pharma-medicine that we cannot even imagine living without it, even though it has only been around for a few generations! See what Mike Adams has to say about this in *The Hidden History of Medicine,* accessible here for free.[195]

Instead of Nature using a "foreign agent" such as a microbe to do the job, notice that today's main sicknesses leading to death are "auto-immune". That is your own body-mind self-destructing, whether it is via cancer, diabetes, lupus, AIDS, M.S., or cardio-vascular degeneration. Have you noticed how someone with diabetes is least likely to cut out sugar and sodas? A stressed person would likewise be even more stressed if he suddenly lost his reason to be stressed. An alcoholic reaches for her next drink even if she knows that she will feel even worse afterwards. And so it is with all forms of self-destruction manifesting as addictions, including destructive and addictive relationships.

What is/are *your* self-destructive addiction/s? *Your* compulsive distractions? Where are *you* being untrue and betraying yourself and your Life Purpose? Before you move on, write the answers here, *now!*

1..

2..

3..

Those who are in greatest denial, in greatest danger, will tragically deny their own addictive tendencies and write nothing above, impatiently reading on to get to the end of the book. So if you are one of them, return to the lines above and don't read on until you have made at least one entry.

Simply blaming modern day pharmaceutical medicine alone is no solution. It takes two to tango, and we must accept responsibility for willingly dancing to their tune, bowing before it, and our addiction to media propaganda. This is the "how and why", out of our weakness of character, we willingly relegate our power and responsibility, happily "selling our souls to the devil".

We need to know what messages we are giving Life. Is your message that you are On Purpose, or that you are lost, off centre, and due for recycling, long before your "expiration" date?

Are you voluntarily relegating your life to faceless organisations that have proved to thrive on poisoning (body, mind, planet)? In other words, do you subscribe to self-destructive thoughts and actions which translate into your own physical destruction? Do you *really* believe that somebody with a degree sponsored by such organisations knows better than you do "for your own good?" Do you *really* believe that manmade drugs are needed to uphold and restore health, and that they are superior to natural remedies to restore our (natural) bodies and minds?

I do not dispute a doctor's highly dedicated training to diagnose physical diseases with the help of pathology departments and technology, or deal with physical trauma/injuries. What I dispute is the focus on illness instead of maximizing health, as well as the denial of the true causes and messages of dis-ease and, leading therefrom, the course of action or remedy prescribed – i.e. "killing the messenger".

Throughout the ages, by contrast, people and organisations genuinely concerned with health and healing (not just profit) have always been aware of the Big Picture, including that we individually, and as a unique part of the Whole, and not some other agent (organisation, environment, human or microbial), are responsible for our health and sickness.

In Ancient Greece, if you were depressed, upset or physically ill, you were not allowed to enter the Polis (City State) and contaminate it, whether it be physically or psychologically. You were directed and would willingly proceed to the Asklepion, where physicians and priests would have you rest and listen to music at specific frequencies specifically composed for you, so as to help you unlock the cause of your issue. Only once *you* (not just your therapist), with the help of oils, bodywork and frequencial rebalancing through sound/healing music, found, understood and transcended the reason for discord within you, could you then proceed to the Polis. This could take minutes, hours, days, or weeks, but took precedence above everything else, as it was known that the thoughts and behaviour of a dis-eased body/mind would bring about undesirable consequences on the individual and society.

Health was not seen as an expense, or even a right, but a personal obligation with full and free support of the *kratos*/State.

This surely played a role for such a tiny space/time/population to set such an unprecedented and unequalled quantum ascent in human consciousness.

Nearly all ancient cultures utilised herbs and natural "soul revealing" or "psychedelic" (ψυχο/pscyho-/=soul, δηλοτικό/ delotico = revealing) substances such as Ergot (*Eleusis* in Ancient Greece); trance-inducing gasses emanating from the Earth (Oracle of Delphi); "magic" mushrooms (notably Nordic Europeans); *ayahuasca*, peyote etc. (the Americas); Cannabis

India; (according to tradition Lord Shiva created it out of His own body); frankincense in the middle east and other substances. *Administered by wise old shamans or priests (male or female, more often female) in great reverence*, these helped us open our minds, get out of the prison of the head, to integrate with our Hearts so as to reconnect with our Source and Purpose.

Even in more recent times, the greatest of people in all fields including nearly (if not) all creative geniuses, great artists and writers, from Francis Bacon (as "Shakespeare"), to visionaries such as Steve Jobs and Richard Branson, have *all* attributed their successes to using psycho-delics, the latter two singing the praises of Cannabis and LSD. .[196]

Modern governments have banned these "drugs", bundling them together with dangerous street drugs (e.g., crack, cocaine, meth etc) which, together with prescribed/"psychiatric" drugs, far from freeing us, drag us screaming and kicking back into the insanity of an imposed reality from which our Hearts yearn to escape. Indeed, many dangerous psychiatric psycho*tropic* (i.e soul *bending*/*distorting*) drugs such as the amphetamine Ritalin®/ Concerta®, which is similar and at least as dangerous as cocaine (adult Ritalin® drug addicts use a much smaller dose than that prescribed to children to reach their "high"), are actively prescribed and even forced onto children for alleged ADD/ADHD.

This is a condition which is diagnosed with alarming frequency, despite the fact that no two doctors or psychiatrists ever agree upon a definition, set of symptoms, or medical test of this alleged "disease". Seasoned research PhD neurologists Drs. Fred Bauchmann and Richard Saul, proclaim ADD/ADHD to be "a fictional disease", an invented excuse to sell drugs to children.[197]

Regarding education, I speak as a post-graduate qualified teacher and counsellor. When you are a child, you are in the "Spring" of your life, full of the joys of Spring. Everything is awe-some and wonder-full and you are an endless source of energy, laughter and goodwill. Then comes school. The e-*duc*-ation system is just that: it takes the young person, squeezes and channels (ducts) her or him into the direction it wants the slaves of the system to go, to produce fodder for the predatory system; "just another brick in the wall" (of our self-built prison), as Pink Floyd so aptly puts it, with the purpose of "matriculation" (initiation into the "matrix").

You may object, saying, "but schooling and education is necessary!", to which I must reply with the historical devolution of education. In ancient Sparta, a Polis (city state) who some may compare to a modern day military "communist" autocracy, children were "educated". The Greek word for "channelled", αγογή/agogi, (agogos=pipe) whereby every boy was "channelled" to be a soldier, finds its equivalent in the Latin "e-duc-cate" (from *ducte*=pipe). Interestingly, the women, who were spared and thus unfettered by this "education", dominated everyday life, despite male figureheads. (As humourously portrayed by the ancient perennial comedy Lysistrata by Aristophanes). However, despite this, the intent of Spartan "agogi" was for the greater social good, and not to serve alien/corporate interests. This was exemplified by King Leonidas and his 300 heroic men who sacrificed their lives, not for Sparta, but for the survival of Athens against the Persian onslaught at Thermopylae.

In Athens, by contrast, all ages went to σχολή/schole, (school) a word which means (place of) leisure. For them, the evolution of a child's (and adult's) intellect was a pleasurable, voluntary ongoing pursuit, where μόρφωση/morphosi, the encouragement of the developement of individual and society was a synergy of individual expression. Only through enthusiam (god/s within) and guided by balance, striving for excellence in pursuit of "knowing thyself" and "questioning the answers" can one/we express our *inherent* αρετή/arête=virtue, fulfilling our Life Purpose, and thus best serve society. A basic Truth long since forgotten.

This was the "schooling" which was created by, and in turn created the society which fathered the arts, sciences, literature, philosophy and is universally hailed as "en-lightening" the world.

However, with the advent of Rome, Caesar subverted the school to become a compulsory institution of indoctrination to serve his interests, by a dehumanising agogi/education, a system whereby your value is based on your blind obedience, and answering rigged questions "correctly" which ruling elites find convenient to implement and impose to this day.

Teaching only obsolete Newtonian science in the Quantum era, disempowering genetics in the age of empowering epigenetics, meaningless mathematics (where the Greeks used mathematics as an empowering link between the physical and metaphysical/spiritual), divisive "history", i.e. propaganda designed to repeat violent history instead of understanding and transcending it, competitive mindsets (divide and rule) instead of win-win synergy, religion which hijacks instead of promoting spirituality etc, so as to "matriculate" us into the *matrix* of blindly obedient automatons. And then we are led to believe that our children, pumped with toxic food and education have a problem when their souls protest, and "need" dangerous amphetamines (prescribed "ADD medication") for "their own good!"

Try to remember your first days at school. Suddenly you stop your spontaneous laughter, your unbounded awe of everything. You become shy and no longer sing for your auntie, or even for yourself. Now that you are " getting big" this is no longer allowed. The child is dead. You have also learned that you are ignorant and stupid and have to do and repeat blindly whatever you are told, and your value depends on how well you do just that. You *don't dare* look out of the window to marvel at the butterfly when the teacher is filling your head with a whole lot of "stuff" (for your own good, of course) out of which your "new identity and self-esteem" is to be formed. ("Good marks, good, clever child. Bad marks, bad child, failure"). In my generation, we were literally "beaten into submission" to robotically "toeing the line" and woe betide anyone having the "audacity" to question.

Nowadays a more sophisticated torture is used: you are no longer acknowledged (even if negatively as a "naughty child,") for overtly or unconsciously resisting educational mind control, but instead "have a psychological problem" called ADD, or ADHD, and as there is no standard definition of either, and indeed no such disease, (I can vouch for that as a parent and a qualified post graduate ex teacher at a "rough" U.K. school) by simple logic, it is thus (ironically) impossible to prove that one does *not* suffer from it. And the "treatment" is the likes of the dangerous amphetamine Methylphenidate (eg Ritalin® and Concerta®) converting you into a subservient moron with good marks. The fact that you have lost your personality, your joy, your Life Purpose, your Soul is seemingly irrelevant (even if you don't believe in the latter). The teacher's (and parent's) job is now much easier. And if Ritalin® leads you to suicide,[198] or "sudden death",[198e] or cancer [198f,] amongst the myriad possible "side-effects", the school may even honour your child's memory with a minute's silence. You don't have to go far to validate what I say about it, it's all in the Ritalin® package insert. Two thirds of its 15 pages is dedicated to numerous "side-effects" including suicide, sudden death and cancer. Did your doctor tell you to study this insert before prescribing it for your child, or have you never even seen this, as the insert is "thoughtfully" removed by the pharmacist? If you still want to go ahead, be it on your head.

We are lost in a world of poisoned environment, poisoned thoughts and poisoned intentions. Every time a messenger, in the form of any physical or psychological discomfort, pops up to guide us, it is fearfully resisted and ruthlessly obliterated. For those of you who are awaiting God/s to talk to them, how do you think He/She/It/they would do it, if not from directing you with happy vs painful consequences as guides/guidelines? Are you expecting God/s to call you on your phone, or maybe to send you an email?

We need to re-dis-cover ourselves; to return to our very Essence, our own Truth, our own Mission. Our whole society, including our equally brainwashed parents (the latter with all misled good intentions), have conspired to keep us total strangers to our Selves. Instead of Knowing Ourselves and being Ourselves, fulfilling our own unique Divine Purpose, we are fearful and resentful moronic slaves, apologetically struggling to fit into an imposed mould.

Now, once again, let's say that you ran the Business of Life on Earth. Would you keep in your employ drugged morons who are not doing the Fun Stuff you gave them to do, but keeping bad company and messing things up for everyone instead, or would you take back the company car (physical body) they have been using and send them back Home, to give them another opportunity to try again in a different time/space from scratch?

The pharmaceutical companies, in addition to ensuring that we are sick, but well enough to stay alive, generating money to keep paying, are integral parts of the system to keep us subservient, in mind and body. To follow and finish up the job done by the companies which through genetic mutation (so-called genetic "modification"),connection with life itself in its various forms is taken away from us, with genetic imperialism via patenting, controlling, confiscating, contaminating our food, living organisms and us.

Antibiotics are logically a major cause of cancer as, besides killing the messenger whilst ignoring the message, as well as compromising our immune system, they are mostly fungi, and by damaging our inner ecology, create ideal conditions for other fungi, including *Candida Albicans* which Dr Tullio Simoncini has identified as the precursor to cancer, as the purpose of a fungus in Nature is to break down and expedite decay.

Fungal infection such as *Candida Albicans* does a number of things. It deprives you of nutrition of the food you eat and literally eats you alive from within. It destroys the living ecology of your gastro intestinal system so that you cannot digest your food properly. It invades your organs, and creates an acid, anaerobic environment which causes decay, which in turn creates an environment for more fungi in a vicious cycle, often ending in cancer, maybe even many years later. Wherever possible avoid antibiotics. Learn about the unparalleled natural antibacterial, anti-fungal and retroviral in this book.

We cannot here go into detail about all medicines and their compromising effect on the body which could directly or indirectly be carcinogenic or compromise your health in various ways. One that "comes up", however, are the "side-effects" of Viagra®;

if your heart is not strong, you can die from a single dose. Thus it may deliver considerably more value than you bargained for by making much more than just your appendage stiff!

Modern pharma medicine plays its treacherous role in our modern "civilization", inculcating helplessness and non-responsibility with respect to our own health, and negating our own unique Purpose, to fit into the plan of an anonymous heartless cabal, being dependent on them as blindly obedient slaves, living and dying for them.

You do not have to be a very skilled doctor to treat an infection pharmaceutically. All you do is take a swab/smear/blood/sputum or other sample from the afflicted person, or the infected site and send it to the lab. Once you have the name of the bug, you simply take out your Mimms directory (the "Holy Book" which gives doctors almost godlike "curative powers" and status), look it up and find the correct antibiotic and dosage. In cases where there is more than one "bug" or the strain is unconfirmed or unknown, you just go for the strongest and most powerful, broad range antibiotic and hope for the best. You should be able to do that for yourself through the internet, but there is an unspoken alliance between medical doctors and pharmaceutical companies: the doctor promotes and prescribes their drugs and in return, the doctor's resources and work becomes privileged, legally enshrined, and not available to "mere mortals".

As we know, medical doctors use similar great ethical wisdom to determine what medicines to prescribe. ..

Enter sexy miniskirted medical rep: "We have this great new drug."
Doctor: "Not interested."
Rep: Bending over the opposite table: "Oh yes you are!"
Doctor, a bit later, whilst closing his trouser zipper: "Excellent drug, will prescribe to my patients!"

While not all medical reps employ this *modus operandi,* the most successful do, and as in all spheres of life there are doctors who, despite medical school brainwashing and subsequent temptations, strive to be ethical, excellent diagnosticians and are compassionate and are of honourable intent, thus performing an integral role in our society. (my own daughter is knowingly studying medicine with a view to becoming a surgeon). It however appears that a disconcerting majority, in this or other ways, does succumb to pharmaceutical sales tactics. How do I know? I have been told this confidentially by not one, but two stunning and highly successful medical reps. But again, don't just rely on my "anecdotal evidence". A google search in April 2014 revealed almost a million results on "drug reps bribing doctors" and of major pharma companies purposefully misrepresenting drugs. GlaxoSmithKline has been repeatedly found guilty, in a court of law, of bribing doctors and persuading them to prescribe an anti-depressant, which is only deemed "safe" for adults, to children, with convictions so far confirmed from the U.S. to China.[199] The fines from such convictions are "petty cash" for such multinationals; a tiny part of the marketing budget.

Ritalin is now also being prescribed to infants, (for whom it was never tested or intended), and in the USA the government has in increasing incidences in an increasing number of states forced children to take Ritalin and other medications against the wishes of the parents, or have them taken away from their families and put under "state care", where they have become "wards of the state" meaning that the State can conduct any medical experimentation it likes on these "human guinea pigs." Unsurprisingly, some have died in such "care."[200]

VACCINES
It's been quite fashionable, the unquestionably "done thing" to go for this and that "shot".

In fact, vaccines are becoming increasingly compulsory for children and entry to schools and other organisations. Rather be shot by a gun, you will at least be spared from potential long term suffering.

Historians, statisticians and top medical researchers with integrity and courage, unswayed by the hype, bribery or threats on their lives have proved beyond any doubt that vaccines have never prevented or turned the tide on any disease, ever; they were all, without exception introduced only after the climax of pandemics such as smallpox and polio, when they had ended their natural cycle and had naturally started to abate.[201] The common factor in the recovery from all epidemics has always been a natural end of the disease's cycle, coupled with a dramatic improvement in hygiene. Bad/good hygiene has proved to be the major cause and cure, respectively, in all epidemics, without exception. If we revert to throwing our excrement out of our windows onto the street as the English did until the Black Plague (possibly onto an unwary passerby's head) see how long it will take for another epidemic to arise.

However in our times, contamination is no longer so obvious. It is insidious in our foods, environment, air and our poisoned thoughts and living styles which we need to redress, and which the pharma mafia have for the most part successfully convinced us to believe are unavoidable problems to be solved and fought by counterpoisoning, with their drugs. An issue amongst others to which this book is dedicated to exposing.

Not only do vaccines not protect our health, but top medical doctors and researchers prove how the toxic contents of vaccines (including mercury and other heavy metals, which in single doses is 25,000 times higher than what is considered "safe"),[202] but have been linked to illnesses, some permanent such as autism, sterility and death, causing far greater affliction, and with much greater frequency than the condition they are supposed to prevent.[203] Even the main line medium NBC Channel aired how HIV virus was found in a major pharmaceutical company vaccine[204].

Furthermore, statements, statistics and recent political history substantiate claims of vaccines as a means of population control,[205] and U.S. government spokesmen are quite blatantly boasting about mind control vaccines by tampering with cerebral DNA.[206]

Before you consider vaccination for you and your children, for instance "Gardsil®," recommended for cervical cancer prevention[207] please do some research first, basing your decision on unadulterated rational scientific historical evidence by *truly* independent, not on "independent" (but actually government/ pharmaceutical sponsored) studies and campaigns or pharma fronts (such as quackwatch.com). You are referred to some more of many other videos and articles from different sources which will hopefully convince you of their dangers,[208] (and by all means do your own research, entering "vaccines" and "autism", AIDS, cancer, deaths, sterilization and almost any other sickness that comes to mind.), including vaccines genetically engineered into food crops planned for release.[209]

Having been convinced of the danger of vaccines, you may feel confused as you find yourself fearfully intimidated by incessant campaigns and misleading statistics by the "authorities who know best". If you don't vaccinate then what protection do you have against disease? The answer is twofold. **Firstly,** vaccinations, further to the dangers they expose you to, do *not* guarantee you immunity to *any* disease. **Secondly**, the *only real protection* we have to *any* disease is a *healthy immune system*. From healthy feelings, thoughts, deeds, and diets; such lifestyles supported by Nature's own apothecary. That is how it always was, and how it always will be.[208d]

Remember that it is in our egoic nature not to want to seek the truth, but to selectively seek out titbits that reinforce what we already believe, no matter how dysfunctional these beliefs may be, and to attack anyone and anything that challenges them. It is so easy and convenient to relegate our responsibilities to "authorities", and then blame a nebulous "them", when, having disempowered and deluded ourselves, things go wrong.

DOCTORS – FROM ROGUES TO HEROES

The problem with medical p*ractices* is that as long as medical doctors do not take personal responsibility for questioning everything which they have been in*doc*trinated (as some do, to their credit) and remain pharma pimps, they are forever *practicing* but never getting it right! Whereas engineers and other professionals are forced to undertake ongoing study to keep up with their professions, in most countries medical doctors are not, and base their "ongoing education" on what drug company sales people "teach" them. Indeed, the problem goes even deeper than this. If you look at medical training worldwide, you will see a "mind control" from the start, with minimal teaching of nutrition, and little or no teaching on promoting and maintaining health, but an emphasis on "drug interventions", supporting Dr Coldwell's aforementioned quote. Most importantly, medicine starts from the dangerous false premise that the symptom or disease is the problem, instead of realising that it is the messenger which will only go away once it or its purpose is understood.

Unlike the traditional Chinese system where one's doctor earned a small monthly stipend from all his patients *except* when they were ill (and thus could not work or generate money) motivating doctors to keep their patients healthy, our system penalizes medics for producing healthy people and rewards them for producing patients. Thus, "sickness maximization" assures profit maximization for the multinational pharmed mafia and doctor. Hermes has tragically long since usurped the control and ethics of the healing profession from Asklepius.

We must not assume that medical doctors are by virtue of their profession inherently any more or less ethical than people in other walks of life, which makes the correct incentives all the more important. By the same token, not every medical doctor is a pharma or ethical sellout. An increasing number of medical doctors are, out of their own initiative, striving to promote and practice "integrative medicine", and are courageously putting themselves at risk of professional ostracism, being struck off the medical roll, imprisonment (eg Dr Simoncini), or even loss of their lives, (with increasing numbers of murders) in addition to those mentioned in this previously referenced free book. [195] Such courageous pioneers for change within and without the medical profession are there to support us, and as sincere, dedicated therapists need and deserve our full support.

An oath to Asklepius is meaningless to the majority of doctors who do not believe in, let alone have reverence for, the Hellenic god of Healing (not medicine, as He is cunningly misconstrued). In order for any oath to be meaningful it should be (or also be) to the god/s of the religion or entity in which one believes or values. Otherwise it is a mockery and a farce.

ALL THAT GLISTENS IS NOT GOLD
(But it Could Save Your Life)

Now you will quite justifiably, ask: what if you contract an infection? It is possible to lose a limb, or even your life from an infection. While it may be all very well to sagely determine the cause, nature and meaning (or message) of the infection, and possibly look at how and why you may have brought the illness or accident upon yourself, or at least made yourself vulnerable to it, this realisation, whilst vitally important, alone cannot help you in such an acute health crisis, where dramatic, instant results are imperative.

Many people will advise you to go to a naturopath, homeopath or other non-medical practitioner. This may work. However, much more expertise is needed and it is far more difficult for a practitioner using natural methods, whose focus is on promoting health rather than simply "attacking the illness", to treat you by addressing the root-cause of your infection, or even the infection itself.

Very few natural therapists have the expertise, knowledge, wisdom, understanding, intuition (or any combinations thereof) for dis-covering and remedying the physical problem (manifestation) as quickly as a course of antibiotics can, as it is much easier and quicker to attack the symptom (infection) directly than treat the cause (compromised immunity).

However, antibiotics are not the only solution. In nearly all cases of infection, there is a far more effective as well as much cheaper solution with no undesirable (so-called "side-") effects.

I have used this with remarkable success, even on people and animals which were at death's door.

When I had an infected tooth abscess which was excruciatingly painful, instead of the prescribed antibiotics, I treated the infection myself by injecting this home-made substance into my gum, every half hour for four hours. The very next morning the swelling was all gone and I felt "normal" again. I am not recommending you do the same and neither am I legally permitted to do so. This is the same substance that saved the entire British Royal Family from the Black Death of 1348 and the Great Plague of 1665 (each of which killed between a third and half of the population of London), what Alexander the Great used for battle wounds and European physicians used before the "Big Pharma" takeover. Now housewives are treating their vaginal thrush, their children's colds and husband's athlete's foot with it. Brave medical doctors in Sweden are using it to treat AIDS,[210] and others to treat cancer.[211]

Its uses are literally endless. It is silver, more specifically colloidal silver.[212] You can get it here,[213] and info and directions as to how, where and when to use it here.[214] However, rather than buy colloidal silver, I would strongly advise you to buy a colloidal silver generator, to save a lot of money, encourage you to use it more, and empower yourself by being able to make whatever quantity you need, whenever you need it. The one I found best in terms of performance, versatility and value for money was this one.[215] As with all the links I give you, visit the book's website often, as these are constantly being updated to ensure that you keep up with the latest and best resources.

Part Three

CLOSING OUR CASE

1. A Cure to Die For — 150
2. The "War Against Cancer" — 155
3. The Heart of the Matter — 159
4. Zooming Out — 162

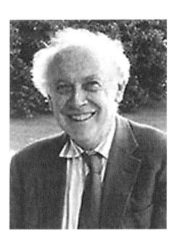

"The National Cancer Program is a bunch of shit."
— **Dr James Watson, 1975, two-time Nobel Laureate, co-discoverer of DNA in 1962**[216]

When you are diagnosed with cancer, you are immediately at the doctor's mercy. He/she will decide whether you will be sent for extremely expensive poisoning which actually causes cancer, usually intravenously (euphemistically known as chemo "therapy"), getting "nuked" i.e. radiation "therapy," radiation being a known carcinogen, or cut (surgery) which often causes metastasis (a spreading or appearance of the cancer elsewhere in the body) or a permutation of two or all three. Is this decision possibly based upon how much your medical aid and you can be made to pay? And why do medical aid schemes not give people an option of (albeit less) money for much cheaper non medical treatment, which would logically save them fortunes. Are they really stupid, or are they getting "kickbacks" at the member's/client's/victim's ultimate expense?

1. A CURE TO DIE FOR

"To sell chemotherapy as a 'therapy' is most likely the biggest deceit in the history of medicine. Whoever masterminded this chemo-torture deserves a monument in hell."
– **Dr Hamer, founder of German New Medicine**[217]

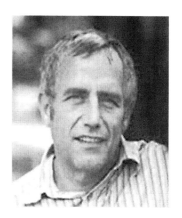

Chemo "therapy" is an extremely cruel and primitive protocol (it's anything but a therapy or treatment) administered on the assumption that the cancerous cells, which are theoretically weaker, will succumb to the poison more than your healthy cells, so that the net result is that a few healthy cells get sacrificed ("collateral damage") to take out more cancerous cells, which is inevitable in any war, but at least you win the war.

In practice, we saw that it does not work that way. Cancer cells are not more vulnerable than healthy cells. To the contrary, they have a hard protective crust around them (the cytochrome P450 enzyme, CYP1B1 which is both a protective crust and carcinogen).[218] Typically, when chemo-"therapy" is initiated, a small decrease in the tumour or evidence of cancer is noted. This is what hooks its victims/"patients". However this does not last long as the cancer usually returns with a vengeance due to your immune system (not on the scan) having being devastated. You, unlike your doctor, now know that the tumour is the symptom and not the cause; and every gardener knows

The TRUTH about CANCER **151**

of a very apt analogy; that if you merely pull out the protruding leaves of the onion weed, this merely serves, not to destroy the weed, but to greatly accelerate the formation of dozens more bulbs underground. If you are not violently ill, doctors see it as a reason to increase the toxicity and/or amount of the "therapy" to your "maximum tolerance" to "get at and defeat the cancer".

However, all that is being achieved is that the cancer is being (albeit invisibly) aggravated, whilst your own immune system and physiology are being destroyed and rendered less capable of standing up to the cancer, and other healthy cells become cancerous from the chemo toxins. Top researchers (free from any monetary interests) agree that most people on chemo "therapy" don't even die from cancer, but from the chemo, from liver and/or kidney failure or "opportunistic infections" from a devastated immune system, but of course this is not divulged or even verified as the deceased's loved ones are left with the "obvious" assumption that "the patient" has succumbed to the cancer (plus they don't have any money left for an expensive, pointless autopsy or any hope of sueing the powerful medical or pharma lobby anyway). Predictably, the pharmaceutical industry has declined any possibility or "usefulness" of such a study.[219c]

An analogy to the logic of chemo-"therapy" is you in a dark room attacked by a pack of wild dogs. I know that you are somewhere in there and try to save you from the beasts by taking pot shots into the darkness with a shot gun. I can judge from the whimpers that I am hitting some dogs, but meanwhile I am filling you with shot as well, while with every yelp more wild dogs rush in to take the place of every dead or dying dog.

What does the medical profession have to say about chemo "therapy"?

"Most cancer patients in this country die of chemotherapy... Chemotherapy does not eliminate breast, colon or lung cancers. This fact has been documented for over a decade. Yet doctors still use chemotherapy for these tumours... Women with breast cancer are likely to die faster with chemo than without it", says

Alan Levin, M.D. (USA), in his book *The Healing of Cancer.*[219] (This applies to any "developed" country and those who can afford this "luxury").

An investigation by the Department of Radiation Oncology, Northern Sydney Cancer Centre, Australia, into the contribution of chemotherapy to five-year survival in 22 major adult malignancies, showed startling results (as "upper limits"): *"The overall contribution of curative and adjuvant cytotoxic chemotherapy to five year survival in adults was estimated to be 2.3% in Australia and 2.1% in the U.S."*[220], as reflected in the U.S. National Library of Medicine website.[221]

On Dr Simoncini's website, polls show that a full *75 percent of doctors say they'd refuse chemotherapy*[223] for themselves and loved ones, due to its ineffectiveness and its devastating side-effects. A similar poll tops 91% for Canadian oncologists.[223c,d]

Professor of medicine, Dr George Mathe, oncologist and past president of the European Organisation for Research and Treatment of Cancer (EORTC) concurred: *"If I were to contract cancer, I would never turn to a certain standard for the therapy of this disease. Cancer patients who stay away from these centres have some chance to make it."* He was accordingly cured of bronchial carcinoma with the help of Hamer's (not so new or German) New German Medicine but, according to GNM.com, continued treating his patients with chemo![224] Is that true? If so, is it because he feared reprisals from the medical establishment? Was it at his patient's insistence? Was he afraid of losing business? Your guess is as good as mine.

Dr EH Willner, M.D., PhD says: *"Established medicine, with little or no evidence to support their barbaric use of these highly toxic drugs, continues to make fortunes while their patients spend their last days vomiting, debilitated, bald-headed and without dignity."*[225]

The official facts are indisputable, and based on the above, and many other references, criticisms of standard medical cancer protocols by prominent medical doctors, researchers and scientists will inevitably lead to the tipping point of their rejection.

So, with mathematical accuracy, how effective is chemotherapy? Let's calculate on the basis that "spontaneous remission", i.e. recovering with no treatment whatsoever, is 14%. 2% − 14% = MINUS 12%! This means that you are almost 12% better off doing NOTHING! In fact, Dr Leonard Coldwell puts spontaneous recovery at almost double the U.S. government figure (of 14%), at 27%.[226] So, using his figures, the chances of recovery without any "conventional medical treatment" then becomes over 29% better! And that is before employing any genuinely therapeutic protocol whatsoever!

Is that good enough for you? And do you know how much the "privilege" of such "therapy" costs? Do you think that this may just be an excellent business proposition for evil people wanting to maximize profit at any monetary and human cost to others?[227] Having said that, I am sure there are many well-meaning but brainwashed, naive medics who are blissfully unaware of these scientifically, statistically verifiable facts. While such people may not be consciously evil, ignorance is no excuse. They are most certainly negligent. No sane conscientious person ever blindly accepts what one is told, particularly when other people place their lives in your hands.

Those seeking further info on chemo "therapy" may at some time want to visit many resources, including these.[227] *But not now.* Let's stay focused and on purpose!

My friend the world famous magician Arthur Reed mentions in his fascinating autobiography, "*The Magic Dragon*"[222], how doctors insisted that a benign old TB scar his wife had, be burned out by radiation "therapy". Immediately thereafter the scar became cancerous, tragically killing her after protracted suffering, leaving him without a wife, companion and partner in his profession and plunging him from fame and prosperity into devastation and debt.

Radiation involves the burning of cancerous tumours using

radioactive sources, which burn much more than the cancerous part, while its intrinsic radioactive nature also **causes** cancer. Surgery is undertaken with your express acknowledgement that the cancer "might spread" *after* the expensive operation which is highly profitable for the hospital and doctors.

As a result of increasingly successful "alternative" cures, together with increased disenchantment with conventional treatments, despite oppressive pro-Big Pharma legislation, pharmaceutical companies, in order to save face have conjured up a new range of expensive "targetted treatments. At a hundred thousand British pounds per session, I know of nobody who has survived more than four sessions. Are you surprised? Based on the Big Pharma track record, can you ever trust them?

Why must you know all of this? The reason is simple. You need to know, **firstly,** what cancer is; **secondly**, how it's caused; **thirdly**, what you can do to prevent it; **fourthly**, about the Cancer Mafia, what it's all about; **fifthly**, to wisen up to future pharma promises, and **most importantly**, how and why you have in fact been programmed to get cancer in the first place! Then and only then will you be empowered and in a position to be response-able for your life and those under your care. Unless you wake up, raise your head, delete and replace the "cancer program", right away, then and only then, can you prevent and treat this condition. So now you know! Its time to act!

Natural, effective and cost-effective cancer treatments are numerous, but this book focuses on prevention. The book on (not treatment, but) healing may follow once there is enough understanding from this book. In fact, if you remain true to the theory and practice of this book, you will not need to buy such book , unless it is for somebody else. However, I am contactable on transcend.apollo@gmail.com for cancer trancendence counselling for those already afflicted. Most significantly though, unless there is an understanding of how and why big money wants you sick, there is no reason, incentive or properly directed motivation to take personal responsibility in this matter.

Cancer is in reality not something to be 'cured', but transcended, and that personal journey is best achieved through personal counselling. I never claim to "cure", but my mission, through personal sessions, group workshops and Skype consultations, is to guide you to a body-mind state where cancer cannot exist, and as a result, you cease to host this condition.

Consult www.cancerfree.cf

2. THE WAR AGAINST CANCER

"Everyone should know that the 'war on cancer' is largely a fraud, and that the major cancer research organisations are derelict in their duties to the people who support them."
– **Linus Pauling PhD, two-time Nobel laureate.**[228]

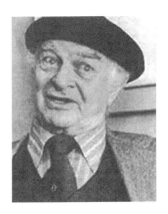

"Intellectually bankrupt, fiscally wasteful and therapeutically useless."
– **Dr. James Watson, two-time Nobel Laureate, on the National Cancer Program**[229]

There is much publicity given to this so-called "war against cancer." Much money is collected. Where does it go? We are told "to the (multinational, multi-trillion dollar) drug companies for 'research'". Cancer incidence has increased and treatment protocols are no less traumatic or more effective. What does this research entail, other than to seek out and "eliminate" anybody with real cures, of which there have been and are, many?

People are encouraged to shave their heads, in sympathy with cancer sufferers, thus further subliminally (unconsciously) fixating the automatic, thoughtless beLIEf that everyone with cancer must/will have chemo-"therapy" and that this is the one and only hope. What sneaky brainwashing! All "good people" *sheepishly* pay to have our heads sheared and wear a pink ribbon in support of breast cancer. How ironically true! Indeed, that *is* supporting breast cancer – unlike a growing minority that is supporting its cure, and more significantly its prevention. And the money collected from the naively well-intentioned brainwashed population, the noble effort, sacrifice and solidarity from you, is used to indoctrinate you even further!

(Read a resume about the "American Cancer Society" and who started it with Dr Burk, PhD and other MD's on engognitive.com, which correctly states "Natural Health is our DNA"[230]).

Women are encouraged to have frequent expensive mammogram scans, whilst researchers have found that women who have mammograms are even MORE, likely to suffer from breast cancer than those that don't. There are two reasons for this: **Firstly,** the mammogram itself is carcinogenic,[231] especially when frequently repeated. Dr Blaylock maintains that each mammogram increases the possibility of cancer by 2%! **Secondly**, the constant thinking and fear of the possibility of breast cancer itself can bring it on via "negative creative" visualisation (the negative placebo or "nocebo" effect, which is evidently much stronger than the "positive" placebo effect). **Thirdly**, and most significantly, only a minority of lumps detected are cancerous, out of which a fifth to a quarter are *non invasive* and would naturally go away, as confirmed in the most significant Norwegian study,[14] whereas the scan, the "nocebo effect" and "treatment" itself can *make* them invasive and fatal. Even some proponents of the scan do not advise it for women under 40 as the carcinogenic affect is worse for younger women on the one hand and on the other, the density of younger breasts make mammogram readings less reliable. Furthermore, neither

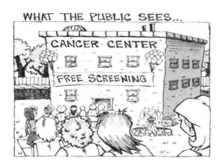
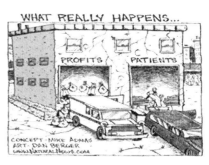

manual examination nor scan is foolproof in terms of finding lumps, cancerous or otherwise, especially with younger women and those with larger and more dense breast tissue.

Interestingly, it is emerging that the most efficient and accurate cancer detectors to date are dogs. Unlike mammograms, and even ultrasound, which seek out lumps, (which may be benign or the result of years of cancerous activity) *dogs can sniff out cancer long before the emergence of tumours or other physical manifestations, whilst ignoring benign lumps.* After dogs were found to have spontaniously discovered cancer in their owners, and warning them, for instance by continuously muzzling and pawing their breasts, dogs are now being trained to detect cancer, with almost 100% accuracy, (far earlier and more accurately than any method created by man) even remotely by sniffing blood, urine and even breath samples!

For those who however trust technology above nature in cancer diagnosis, and have been fearfully conditioned into having to be screened, I would suggest neither the mammogram nor the somewhat safer ultrasound scan/sonogram, which both seek out lumps. Instead insist on thermography. This method does not involve squeezing the breasts (as with mammograms) and, like the dog, detects cancer at far earlier stages than the two aformentioned ways, as it does not seek out lumps, but rather heat anomalies implying *carcinogenic processes which happen long before the formation of lumps.* Indeed, finding a cancerous lump is in a very real sense, already "too late".

Mammograms can thus be seen to be nothing else but a lucrative cancer patient recruitment protocol.

In short, the "War against Cancer", like the "War against Drugs", "Fighting for Peace" and the alcohol "Prohibition" of the 1930s are all, as the hippies of the 1960s said, like "f@#king for Virginity", an evil plot to perpetuate exactly what they supposedly oppose. *What you focus on always gets bigger.* Resistance is a form of focusing on a problem instead of a solution, which is why *"what you resist, persists"* (CG Jung). The proponents of the "wars on cancer, terrorism, crime" etc know this only too well, and thus they enlist our time, energy, emotions and efforts to perpetuate such problems, whilst they cash in at our expense.

The latest version of the "war against cancer" is the MEMS (micro electromechanical system) microchip. For years it has been in the interests of a small minority to microchip everybody, and what better way to do this than to make people want it, be willing to pay for it and even beg for it? And so it is with the MEMS microchip technology.[232] Barely larger than a grain of rice, this chip is easily implanted under the skin, and monitors your health on a continuous, nonstop basis, doing away with expensive and time-consuming medical visits and tests and sending the results to your computer, your phone, your doctor, and.....?

What they don't tell you is that the MEMS also sends details of your health, your emotions, your whereabouts, everything about you, to other people and places you do not know. Also, and most significantly, they don't tell you that it is not just a transmitter, but also a receiver, capable of releasing drugs and affecting changes in your body remotely, without your knowledge, let alone permission, and even killing you. We are already followed and have our privacy intruded through our cellphones, GPSs, computer IPs (internet protocol address), RFID (radio frequency identification), microchipped "I.D documents",passports, etc. Do you really want to willingly assist in putting total control of your health, mind, and life into the hands of unknown people and interest groups? I don't. I would rather take personal responsibility to live healthily, and to the fullest extent possible, freely, independently, privately, and fearlessly.

Removing cancer from our lives is done in a completely different way to monitoring and intervention by others, and more specifically, mindless subservience to a system which by its very nature is predatory and itself cancerous.

Firstly, the emphasis should not be on fighting, nor even on cancer (nor Ebola,Zika nor anything else). It cannot be repeated enough: What you focus on always increases. Whether you love or fear/hate something, your time, attention, thought and energy empowers and manifests it. That is why emphasis needs instead to be placed on vibrant, not just "good", but radiant health.

Secondly, this state of health is achieved, not by passively waiting and going for screening, but by positive, active awareness of our thoughts, and proactivity in our deeds. Don't preach, but be a living example, and before you know it, there will be enough of us, through the so called "100th monkey effect", to change the world. Your commitment to this started with buying this book. Maybe this book should have simply been titled *"Optimizing Joy and Health in your Life"* but unfortunately, few people relate to this as the ultimate defence against cancer. A "side-effect", if you will.

Thirdly, the realization that this is to be done on an individual, community, national and global level, in order to create the environment in which cancer will no longer have a place, from the personal (microcosmic) level to the global (macrocosmic) level of planetary health, as presented in our closing chapter.

Let the "International Cancer Awareness Campaigns/Days" be replaced with "International Health Awareness Campaigns/Days".

3. THE HEART OF THE MATTER

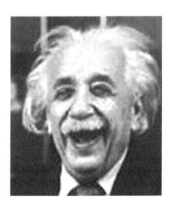

"The intuitive mind is a sacred gift and the rational mind is a faithful servant. We have created a society that honours the servant and has forgotten the gift." [233]
– **Albert Einstein**[233]

If you take a purely "left-brained", intellectual approach to everything, everything will be working, just as it was, with perfect efficiency and totally meaninglessly until life overtakes the old and it collapses and dies, taking you with it. It begs the question: Is there life *before* death? In this case, the answer can only be an emphatic No! You live to work, and work to live. What's the point?

If on the other hand, you take a purely emotional, "right-brained" approach to life, everything is constantly in turmoil, as you allow circumstances (circum=around; stances=standing,or things around you) and other people in your life to take you from high crests to the lowest troughs on stormy waters. Nothing works consistently, especially you, as you rush around lighting and putting out fires. There certainly is life before death, but is it worth all that stress and trauma?

Predominantly "left brained" people are addicted to escapism by cleverly fabricated intellectual denial and detachment, whilst "right brained" people are addicted to fearful attachment, imagining things that dont exist, exaggeration and dramatization. Both "thrive"/are addicted to distractions of the media, consumerism, identification with belief systems, hero worship, etc. Can you see from what we have learnt that both extremes are breeding grounds for cancer? Neither are *proactive*, but (unconscious/ programmed) default reactions to fear – the former by denial, the latter by indulgence. So what is the alternative?

Does it not make sense to suggest returning to the one and only part of the body which never succumbs to cancer? This is why the most significant thing you can do to secure optimum health is to return to your own True (Heart) Centre.

Every morning upon arising and preferably before sleeping, give yourself (and partner) 15 minutes of silent meditation. If you like, you can have gentle music blending into an arousing wakeup rather than a simple rude alarm. These 15 minutes of centreing will most certainly be worth much more than the 15 or even 30 minutes of sleep foregone, as it is busy and confused thoughts, not what you do, which cause greatest turmoil and exhaustion.
You can find numerous free delta-wave binaural (headphones essential), isochronic (headphones not needed) and iso/binaural soundtracks on YouTube. Delta waves are the second slowest (lowest frequency) brainwaves after Epsilon waves.

These are most helpful in helping even the most busy mind enter a slumbersome state. It is well worth your while seeking out one or more which work for you.These sound tracks can be in the form of a pure tone, set to music, and/or accompanied by a guided meditation or sleep hypnosis. Likewise, different frequencies can facilitate whatever mindstate serves you at any time.

Delta waves are best at bed-time, whilst the slightly higher frequency theta waves are best for day-time meditation. The next frequency up, alpha, is ideal for creativity, work and study. The higher beta and highest gamma brainwaves, to which we have become addicted, naturally occur for "fight or flight" situations, invoking the primitive part of our brain, flooding us with stress hormones, starving our vital organs of oxygenated blood, and when continuous is the main cause of sicknes and premature death today. One way or another. Directly or indirectly.

Alternatively, meditate to, and/or experiment with playing in the background at various times, solfeggio frequencies of 396Hz, 417Hz, 432Hz, 528Hz, 639Hz, 741Hz, 825Hz, or 963Hz, also freely available on Youtube.These correspond to diffent psycho/physical centres (or 'chakras') which are in turn linked to different glands in the endocrine system. Trust your feelings. You will find which frequency/ies and tracks work best for you at any time, and commit this time daily to yourself. For more information visit this free and informative site about the specific benefits of each frequency, as well as other interesting resources.[234] The 528Hz tone is said by some to be the most important frequency, as the Heart, miracle and DNA-repair tone, while others promote the Universal Pythagorean 432Hz frequency. Experiment for yourself! To most people (including me), this frequency may sound irritating at first, but this response soon yields to a sense of wellbeing The initial irritation may merely be ego resistance to its loss of control as we link with our "Higher Selves".

Healing vs harming frequencies is a study in itself which has for the last millenia been withheld from the general population, whilst having been used since ancient times for healing in the Asclepia and destructively in the biblical account to bring down the walls of Jericho. Sound and light frequencies are quickly regaining their place in health maintenance and healing with their "rediscovery" through quantum therory, in tandem with a deeper understanding of the highly sophisticated Pythagorean teachings and healing techniques used in the Asclepia and Ayurveda ("*ayur*" corresponds with the Greek "*aήp*"/*aer*, or aetheric resonance, the "first cause" of life)

Using something simple and basic as delta waves (binaural and/or isochronic) or a solfeggio frequency which feels right for you will ensure that you have a restful night's sleep and start the day in a powerfully centred, but serene, competent and balanced way; as *You*. (Before family, work and society claim you for their own ends). There is nothing in the world more precious than this.

Using a computer analogy, the heart is the motherboard and the head is the processor. Of all messages between the heart and brain, 90% originate from the heart.[235] The electromagnetic field radiated from the Heart is also about 50 times stronger than that radiated from the brain. The heart is also the source of a unique "universal/spiritual" non-electromagnetic-type longitudinal wave energy that travels faster than "Maxwell's Constant", the speed of light (which is a transverse, electromagnetic wave). [236]

I restrain myself from the temptation of saying a lot more in this book about the heart now, other than to mention that recent science has proved that the heart is a lot more than a mere pump, and that ancient wisdom regarding the primacy of this organ, physically and spiritually, is being scientifically proven here,[236] amongst numerous other sources. This is notwithstanding that from a spiritual energy perspective, the "Heart Centre/chakra", while including the physical heart, is in fact not centred on the physical heart itself, but on the nearby thymus gland, which (surprise-surprise!) governs the immune system.

Recommending connection to the heart and harmonizing it with your head is easier said than done, not because it is inherently difficult, but because it needs dedication and perseverance to overcome habitual behaviour in this respect.

This can be further facilitated by an instrument which I use,[237] namely a cardiac biofeedback device, smaller, cheaper, quicker and far more effective than any of the expensive and difficult to use brain biofeedback systems in medical laboratories. I have found its benefits in all areas of life to far exceed its maker's claims, which are constrained to comply with the law.

Knowledge and thinking are useful tools, but nothing and nobody can replace your Inner Guidance, or teach you how to be the real *You*. If you were to take only one thing from this book, let it be this. If we quieten our minds from distraction and tune into our own Divine Purpose, the Whole Universe will conspire to support us, with unfailing, optimal Health, with "all else added unto us".

4. ZOOMING OUT: YOU, CANCER, AND THE BIG PICTURE

"The Macrocosm is in the Microcosm"

"As above, so below". "Above", here, refers to "Higher Resonances", or the spiritual plane, and "below", the material plane. "Above" and "below" should not be taken as value judgments of "superiority/inferiority" or "good/bad", but more like the "head" and "tail" of a coin. In order for the coin to manifest physically, it must have a "tail side" opposing the figurehead in whose name the coin was created.

"As within, so without". "Within" on a personal level is our own emotional and rational state of mind, which in turn affects our relationship with life, other people, our environment and indeed, the world itself. "Within" starts at our thoughts and feelings, which directly affects the material world at the quantum level (as conclusively and repeatedly proven, for instance in the twin slit light experiment[238]) which outwardly affects water as we have seen,(even by passive observation!)
- which outwardly affects our hormones and body chemicals,
- which outwardly affect our cells,
- which is then reflected in our overall health,

• which, in turn, affects our behaviour and the world we create.

At this point we can either *re-act* to the environment and circumstances we have created, directly or indirectly (as individuals or as the human race), thus creating a vicious circle, or we can respond – in other words, act response-ably. To what extent are you (unconsciously) re-actionary, and to what extent (consciously) response-able ("responsible") and pro-active? A victim or a creator? To be the guineapig of, or the change you want to see in the world?

If you are not experiencing cancer now, you now have no reason to worriedly lie in wait for it, passively taking tests (like radioactive carcinogenic mammograms) and hoping for the best.

You now know the causes of cancer, and you know why it proliferates.

You now also know how the cancer business operates.

But most importantly, you know the practical steps to release yourself from the cancer body-mind programming, so as to reclaim mastery of your life and your health.

You can now focus, not on the fear as to whether you may have the "bad luck" of "being a victim" to cancer, but rather to proactively dedicate yourself to maximizing radiant health in all areas of your life, from how you perceive yourself and your life/circumstances/world, to attitude and behaviour, first for yourself and thereafter (because you are functioning from Purpose) for people, society, and Earth Herself. Your love for yourself and the world are ultimately but two aspects of the same thing (or "coin").

Microcosmic malevolent ("bad" or "ill intentioned", deadly) cell proliferation (cancer) in our bodies we now know cannot be separated from the macrocosmic cancer of a disastrous and toxic human contamination of our Great Mother Earth. In reality, the one is merely a reflection of the other.

Indeed, an aerial, or macroscopic view of the destructive and overwhelming way in which humans have overrun the planet, as host-destroying parasites which eventually kill their host and thus ultimately bring about their own demise, looks almost identical, by analogy to cancerous human tissue, as mentioned.[240]

To quote a pet phrase of Dr Bruce Lipton, "Every cell is a little me".

In the same way, our world is composed of and determined by us, and just as each cell is a "little me", we are a "little world"; however, we now have the conscious awareness to proactively choose to make a healthy difference.

There are less of us in the world (7 billion) than there are cells in our bodies, estimated at around 75 *trillion*. This immediately makes our potential effect on the world over 10 000 times greater than the effect single cells in our bodies have on us.[239] However, this effect is directly proportional to our emotional state. If we come from a state of fear, we will merely reactively purpetuate a sick state, but to the degree that we come from the empowering state of Love, we can and do change it for the better, both directly and physically, as well as subtly and energetically. The good news is that a 'positive mind state is far more powerful than a negative one, as it is in harmony with the Universe/God/s rather than from a fearfully detatched little ego state.

Environmental gedradation applies to some extent to all civilizations (where "civil" refers to "city dwelling societies") and most especially modern Man, with our religious alienation from nature and our self-appointed "ownership" and exploitative "dominion" of the Earth, our greed and our misused technology. Only so-called "primitive people" lived integrated with and in harmony with nature . The challenge is upon us, not to reject technology, or try to "reverse" civilization, but to implement it in such a way that we may once again live in harmony with nature and, instead of creating waste and destruction, becoming a congruent and consciously participative part of its evolution. What could be referred to as the "return of the prodigal son", or humanity having completed a full circle and finally arrived back to its source, this time out of awareness and free choice.

So how does this affect you as an individual? As a former cancer candidate? Whilst, on the one hand, our physical, mental

166 The TRUTH about CANCER

and emotional environment poisons us, it is we (as a race and as individuals) who have created environmental destruction by our own poisoned beliefs, thoughts, and intentions in the first place.

Just as we cannot be truly healthy unless our relationship with our human mother is healthy, or at least reconciled, it is essential that our relationship with Mother Earth, in whose Womb and Embrace we are given this physical life (until the time we return our bodies back to Her), is similarly reconciled. It is impossible for humans to be cancerous cells heading rapidly towards overloading and killing Earth without the same cancerous symptoms reflecting and manifesting in us as well. It's nothing "personal"; in fact it's totally impersonal. Give it a logical, scientific label ("cause-and-effect") or a religious label ("karma"/ as you sow, so shall you reap/kismet, etc), it makes no difference, but that is what it is.

That is why we now need to work equally "without" (i.e., outside of ourselves, wherever we find ourselves) and "within" to heal the results of cancerous thinking in the past, by becoming aware, taking responsibility, choosing to be "response-able" for our personal negative impact on the environment and, in our own way, take an active role in changing it. This includes such "outward" actions as recycling, boycotting environmentally unfriendly products, pursuing cleaner, less wasteful technologies and lifestyles, participating in clean-ups, etc., according to our individual position and ability. Simultaneously with these outward-facing actions, changing us from being a human cancer cell, and part of the problem, to being part of the solution, we undergo an internal transformation, which heals our own internal proclivity for cancer (and vice versa). You and I are a part of the cancerous human race, just like anyone else, unless we consciously choose otherwise. Each one of us can decide whether to succumb to this unconscious, fear-based cancerous mass of socially engeneered humanity, (mindless following as part of the problem) or to be a self-aware, conscious, healthy individual of noble intent, and thus becoming a vitally vibrant "cell"(leading as part of the solution).

Do we align with a fear-based, dis-integrative mortal ego state, or with an integrative, omnipotent and immortal universe? When

Jesus was convicted of blasphemy, claiming to be the "Son of God", he reminded his judges that, according to their own Mosaic Law, humankind was told by the 'Lord' that "we are (all) gods" (John 10:34; Ps. 82.6). The part of us (egoic or godly) with which we identify determines our feelings, thoughts and actions, which in turn determines the health of ourselves and our world. Long before that, the Hellenes also held that we mortals are equivalent to gods, refusing to bow before anyone, mortal or immortal, honouring their gods not by cowering, or "bowing before", but by standing upright with arms outstretched and palms open. The Greek word for "human", άνθρωπος/*anthropos* literally means "upward looking", for it is indeed our outlook in life which determines our thoughts, our, character our actions, and ourselves. Risng joyfully towards, inspired by, and not cowering fearfully before the Divine.

Being "godly" or "holy" means connection and allegiance to the One, Omnipotent "Whole", and for access to that infinite power we need to cast our fearful little egos aside and *Be* the Connecting Love of One *in practice*, not just in doctrine or theory.

A scientist may well correctly say that, at the end of the day, we are nothing more than a bunch of photons resonating in a magnetic field. A spiritual teacher would not object, but merely continue to point out that it is exactly this field of energy which is behind our whole universe, and which acts in perfect unison, what has been referred to as the aetheric "Supreme Unified Beingness" Γ"Οντος Ον by the Ancient Hellenes (Greeks), the "Great Spirit" by the American "Indians", or simply "God" by most of my readers. The microcosm and macrocosm are thus one and the same, reflections of one another, the "Unified Field"

We seem to have forgotten that. We have become *dis-integrated,* lost our identity, sense of belonging, our "membership" of the Great "One", thousands of years ago. Isn't it time we *re-membered* ourselves?

Just as an eagle brought up amongst chickens will live the life of a chicken, so a human brought up in a world of "humanoid sheep" ("sheeple") will always be a sheep, unless each one of us courageously makes a conscious choice to wake up. This needs courage, commitment, persistence and perseverance. To quote Ghandi, "First they ignore you, then they ridicule you, then they fight you, then you win!" (And eventually they build a monument to you). In support of taking your own stand in life, remember Krishnamurti's words: "It is no measure of health to be well adjusted to a profoundly sick society."

The true "leap of faith" is to find this "Divine Connection Within," and not "out there" in the many "beLIEf systems" which seek to disempower, divide, control and rule us.

It is no big deal to deny the dark and seek out the light. Anybody can do that. But it takes a Great Soul to confront the darkness and *Be* the Light! And everyone is hiding a "Great Soul" but few have the awareness or courage to connect with it! How about you, now?

It is not complicated. It starts and ends with Intent. It is no more or less accessible to anyone, regardless of place, time, age, sex, wealth etc. Neither is it easy. But the choice is between what religions describe as "heaven" or "hell", except that these options are in the *here and now* rather than in some afterlife.

What about religion? Well, firstly, spirituality and religion are not the same. Religion is a societal doctrine demanding blind faith in a conditioned belief over your own experiential reason, in most cases initially violently imposed until it becomes unconsciously imprinted and fearfully unquestioned through the generations. Our purpose here is not to enter into a religious discourse, but to transcend it.

If your religion is a way of connecting you to All of Humanity, to Life itself, identifying with Love, accepting and integrating everything and everybody, whilst honouring your own views as well as respecting those of others, and you live in childlike fascination; if you see yourself and your society as a unique but integral part of the whole and that "heaven or hell" is a state we can choose in the here and now, not in an afterlife, then your religion, by its nature, is spiritual.

If, however, you believe that your religion, race, beliefs, tradition, ancestry, heritage, nation, scientific/social/economic/political or other ideology, or category is exclusive, separate, "different" or superior in any way, then your religion (whether it is based on a belief in God/gods, doctrines, money, science, materialism etc.) is disconnecting you from Reality – material, spiritual, or otherwise. This, in turn, imprisons you in your self-righteous ego (programmed by others) merely as a robotic, easily manipulated tool used by a small minority to divide and rule humanity with tragic consequences for all. Flush it away! Don't let parents, family, community, social institutions ("the flock") keep you imprisoned!

One can compare these two conceptions of "religion" to healthy *vs* unhealthy sexual behaviour, where (on the one hand) true connection is made with another in the fullest sense in a mutually empowering relationship (healthy); and (on the other hand), locking yourself up to solitarily indulge in pornography (unhealthy). Where the one brings true connection, the other brings separation and self-delusory gratification that is not connective, but strongly disconnective, making you withdraw from any situation or possibility of a meaningful connective relationship – with others, or with the Divine, but primarily and ultimately, with yourself.

Wake up! We are all in this together! Cancer happens when an organism, whether it is our body, society, or the world is not integrated, connected or in harmony. Whenever there is imbalance or internal strife, the cancer, as colonisers do, now rules by default. It is no "coincidence" that cancer is proliferating now. The world is becoming One. Globalisation is here, like it or not. The question is: How? Will it be a manipulated, conflicting world, forcefully dominated and homogenised by a faceless, ominous seemingly almighty cancerous, "New World Order?" Or will we cherish our differences, learn from and share with one another, seek to know and love ourselves and each other, free from cancer, both with-in and with-out as a joyfully Synergizing, Integrated World, not only sustainable but creatively and purposefully evolving?

You are either a part of the problem (cancer), or part of the solution. Choose now!

I invite you to accept the challenge.

Raise your Head up High! Accept Yourself! Be Yourself! Question the Answers! Ask the "forbidden" questions! Courageously challenge and confront your fears! Blaze the path of (inner) Joy, instead of desperately seeking and pursuing (outer) happiness! Laugh loudly, daily! Heal Yourself and Heal the World!

Your/Our lives, our children's lives and our world is literally in your hands!

Thank you for joining me on this adventure! Stay in touch with developments on the site **www.cancerfree.cf** – Register here [241] for news, updates, helpful articles, and occasional offers, including priority on future events, and first views on future books.

Wishes and blessings for a Life of Great Joy, Profound Meaning and that each one of you find and fulfil your Life Purpose for the Benefit of All.

Whilst this book gives a clear roadmap for leaving the cancer trap and healthy living, it was with difficulty that I resisted including some "higher level" information, which I can share in upcoming books on the transcendence of cancer and other issues, once this one is accepted, integrated and acted upon.

Whilst a truly holistic book on transcending cancer is sorely needed and will be written, it cannot replace personalised Wellness and Cancer Transcendence Coaching for international clients on Skype and which can be arranged on cancerfree.cf or by emailing transcend.apollo@gmail.com

Facebook users can be updated on Fotini Economou's most informative facebook group:

"The Truth about Cancer, Prevention is Better than Cure."

ALL PHYSICIANS!

Remember, your oath is to heal, and at least not harm **people!**

You have a sacred obligation and responsibility to those who trust you with their lives! Not to multinational corporations, or their bribes, 'education' and large 'kickbacks'! I have been approached by numerous physicians (medical & otherwise)   for physician's training. No names divulged. Be independently informed, to make informed decisions. Give your patients informed choices!

PS.

For Skype sessions, workshops, or embarking on a profound and courageous, shamanic voyage of Self Discovery, on your own, or in an intimate group, of breaking the mould (in both senses of the word) and Knowing Thyself, as did our ancient forefathers, feel welcome to contact me on transcend.apollo@gmail.com, or my wonderful staff, networkers and associates

Book Website and updates: www.cancerfree.cf
email author on site or on: booksthatheal@gmail.com
skype: by arrangement

Other upcoming titles:
"PANARCHY, the Ultimate Freedom for You and the
 World"
The Controversial Eye-opener!
Booklets:
* "GOOD PEOPLE NEVER SAY "PLEASE"
* "LOVE IS (not what you think)"
* "YOU ARE NOT WHO YOU THINK (and I can prove it)"

Inspirational Fiction
  * **The Tokolosh, Great Heart and You(c)**
  * **Thembela's Odyssey(c)**

Subscribe to the newsletter on *http://cancerfree.cf* which will always provide interesting information, answers to your questions, articles and updates for FREE as well as provide benefits, discounts and other offers from time to time. ●

Part Four

Bibliography / References

Rerefence seeking tips:
Some online references may have moved or been hacked or deleted.
If you don't find your reference, try:
1 – Searching on the site's home page (remove letters after the .com, .org etc)
2 – You tube videos may have been removed and reposted
3 – Search for article name or topic:"good gopher" seems a promising search engine for the future, influenced by popular vote, not corporate interest.
4 – Take the initiative and do your own research!

CANCER & YOU

1 – Official Statistics
a. Prediction & Prevention
http://www.webmd.com/cancer/news/20030407/global-cancer-rates-to-rise-50-by-2020
b. http://www.who.int/mediacentre/news/releases/2003/pr27/en/

2 – 70% in 20 yrs
a. The Guardian: http://www.theguardian.com/society/2014/feb/03/worldwide-cancer-cases-soar-next-20-years
b. The Independent: http://www.independent.co.uk/life-style/health-and-families/health-news/new-cases-could- rise-by-70-per-cent-in-20- years-9104983.html
c. Denver Post: http://www.denverpost.com/fitness/ci_25051699/cancer-cases-expected-increase-70-over-next-20
d. PolicyMic: http://www.policymic.com/articles/81169/global-cancer-rates-expected-to-soar-by-70-over-next-20-years-here-s-why

3 – Depopulation
a. http://www.prisonplanet.com/the-population-reduction-agenda-for-

dummies.html (if unavailable, do "depopulation" search)
b. (2h6m) https://www.youtube.com/watch?v=dUWByt813fA
c. WTF! Bill Gates depolulation plans (typo on original)
https://www.youtube.com/watch?v=3TyAJZVARPw
d. Ebola article: https://www.lifesitenews.com/news/fbi-interested-in-texas-doomsday-ecologist-who-said-ebola-the-solution-to-h

4. Dr Coldwell stopped cancer in family. **Video**
https://www.youtube.com/watch?v=uWQ8zFeLaIc

4A Dr Coldwell, personal determination. **Video**
The surprising true causes of cancer: (5m) https://www.youtube.com/watch?v=hX49Q1A8_PE

4B Dr Coldwell, book **"The Only Answer to Cancer"**
http://tinyurl.com/nrx5eb6

5. Bruce Lipton video,
Epigenetics, the Science of Empowerment
a. Epigenetics (shortest) 7m https://www.youtube.com/watch?v=BjjvimJRevQ (intermittent)
b. (short)15m https://www.youtube.com/watch?v=YBS7ju6O1xQ
c. (medium) 42m https://www.youtube.com/watch?v=kqG5TagD0uU (intermittent)
d. Epigenetics (long) 1h10m https://www.youtube.com/watch?v=_xz1HrGG8cc
e. Epigenetics (longer) 2h39m https://www.youtube.com/watch?v=c_kwbHpBKEo

5B Dr Lipton book: – The Biology of Belief:
Unleashing the Power of Consciousness, Matter, & Miracles.
By-a-seasoned academic! Read it! You will never be the same!
http://tinyurl.com/p3udztw

6. – Dr Sam Epstein and other powerful quotes:
http://www.whale.to/cancer/quotes.html
Articles by Dr Epstein: http://www.healthy-communications.com/epstein'spage.html (intermittent)

7. – Dr Sanford D.C.B.S. 98% lifestyle
(internet reference expired, but his site is: www.adjustdallas.com)

QUESTIONS DEMANDING ANSWERS

8. Farben/Hoesht/Bayer 1
a. http://www4.dr-rath-foundation.org/PHARMACEUTICAL_BUSINESS/history_of_the_pharmaceutical_industry.htm

b. http://www.whale.to/b/nazi_allopathy.html
c. http://www.corporatewatch.org/id=317
(if page removed omit id=317)
d. http://www.relay-of-life.org/speech/speech.html
e. Monsanto = fda and govt : http://www.redicecreations.com/specialreports/monsanto.html (search "monsanto" on site if this page expires)
f. Take a Stand! Sign Movement of Life: http://www.movement-of-life.org. (search "take action")
http://www.movementoflife.org/takeaction?RNAL&pk_kwd=RELAYOFLIFE130924

9. **Selective Seratonin Reuptake Inhibitors & Safe Alternatives** (eg Prozac®, Zoloft®) vs serotonin & dopamine increase with cannabis
a. Why Antidepressents Are No Better Than Placebos: ttp://www.newsweek.com/why-antidepressants-are-no-better-placebos-71111
b. Why its Better to Have a Mind than a Brain. Deepak Chopra
http://www.huffingtonpost.com/deepak-chopra/why-its-better-to-have-a_b_471278.html
http://www.oprah.com/spirit/Why-Its-Better-to-Have-a-Mind-Than-a-Brain
c. HIGHLY RECOMMENDED: Peter Gotzsche, Cochrane Collaboration:Deadly Medicines and Organized Crime (16m)
https://www.youtube.com/watch?v=VIIQVII7DYY#t=43
Cannabis
d. cannabis is a natural safer, cheaper and more effective treatment for ADHD
http://www.chanvre-info.ch/info/en/Cannabis-as-a-medical-treatment.html (if page expires, simply enter www.chanvre-info.ch)
e. Dr Beardman, Dr C Jensen:
http://www.truthonpot.com/2013/04/01/medical-marijuana-and-adhd-the-facts/
Cannabis and ADD/ADHD
e. http://www.leafly.com/news/health/cannabis-and-addadhd
e1. http://www.leafly.com/knowledge-center/medical-resources/cannabis-and-addadhd

10. **Sceletium tortuosum**
a. www.sceletium.org
b. **Order Sceletium Tortuosum/kanna** http://tinyurl.com/nutjzk
or at http://cancerfree.cf
c. http://en.wikipedia.org/wiki/Sceletium_tortuosum

11. **Death by medicine, by Dr Gary Null PhD, Dr Dorothy Smith**

PhD and 3MD's

a. http://www.webdc.com/pdfs/deathbymedicine.pdf   or alternatively, http://www.lef.org/magazine/2004/3/awsi_death/Page-01 Bhttp://www.whale.to/a/null9.htmlUY the full BOOK!... http://tinyurl.com/omy837l

b. Also: **Death by Prescription: Dr Ray Strand:** http://tinyurl.com/oqej8j8

c.. Dr Null's article discussed by Bruce Lipton: The Biology of Belief: (13th minute of 2h31m video

12. – Dr Coldwell's book:-"Instinct Based Medicine: How to Survive your Illness & Your Doctor"
Disillusioned doctors are the biggest opponents of today's medicine. http://tinyurl.com/qzeddnb

13. – Nat Med Libr 5 to 3 tr surv rates & survival rates
Nhi&Austr sites – see 14

14. – Norwegian Breast Cancer Study on U.S. National Library of Medicine.
Spontaneous remission of mammography detected invasive breast cancers

a. spontaneous healing observed for hundreds of thousands of years "an indisputable fact": http://www.ncbi.nlm.nih.gov/pmc/articles/PMC3312698/

b. Dartmouth Med School. "quite common": http://dartmed.dartmouth.edu/spring09/html/disc_remission.php http://www.curezone.org/forums/am.asp?i=1782306

c. http://www.dailymail.co.uk/health/article-1172211/The-miracle-survivor-I-given-months-live-terminal-cancer-vanished.html

d. "Shocking Study". http://talesfromtheconspiratum.com/2013/11/25/shocking-study-spontaneous-remission-of-breast-cancer-found-to-be-common/ (site repeatedly attacked)

e. less testing=less cancer: http://www.futurepundit.com/archives/005744.html

15. – Steve Jobs – death attributed to "conventional treatments" http://www.naturalnews.com/033793_steve_jobs_chemotherapy.Html
from dominating google search, now a mysterious absence of results

Part I **3. OUR OBJECTIVE**
        4. WHAT IS CANCER?

16. – Metastasis slightly more likely after breast surgery

http://www.sabcs.org/PressReleases/
Documents/2013/8441ed234d66e516.pdf

17. Moritz book reference
Cancer Is Not a Disease – It's a Survival Mechanism. A total
paradigm shift on cancer! http://tinyurl.com/pwkyewq

18. de Martini book: *The Value Factor*
http://tinyurl.com/kpkuno8

19 Cancer & Earth
a. http://www.youtube.com/watch?v=C0R6EvtGnoE
b. **Dr Warren Hern:**
http://www.drhern.com/pdfs/humancancerplanet.pdf
c. **KentMcDougall:**
(I do not subscribe to the doctrine of this church, but this
article has scientific merit and is very pertinent:)
http://www.churchofeuthanasia.org/e-sermons/humcan.html
d. **Excellent all round article:**
http://www.kospublishing.com/html/cancer.html

Part I 5. THE BUSINESS OF CANCER

20. Money Ponzi scheme
a. http://www.globalresearch.ca/25-fast-facts-about-the-federal-
reserve-biggest-ponzi-scheme-in-world – history/5373609
b. (4m) https://www.youtube.com/watch?v=WhwUiBGxufM
c. Money as debt: excellent animation, easy to understand (47m)
https://www.youtube.com/watch?v=jqvKjsIxT_8
d. The Biggest scam... (30m)
https://www.youtube.com/watch?v=iFDe5kUUyT0

21 CIA runs worldwide drugs
a. Intro: The CIA's Involvement in Drug Trafficking: (9m)
https://www.youtube.com/watch?v=5b6kf5PIzX4
b. Morbid Addiction. CIA and the Drug Trade (19m)
https://www.youtube.com/watch?v=_9bhFu-dmB0
c. The phoney drug war: (16m)
https://www.youtube.com/watch?v=qJkFZ4W4bjg
d. (11m) https://www.youtube.com/watch?v=0LqDjk8vhyc
e. CIA drug trafficking
https://www.youtube.com/watch?v=2M3I9X3gR2A
f. Phony drug war.(16m)
https://www.youtube.com/watch?v=qJkFZ4W4bjg
g. CIA drug consp(1h46m)
https://www.youtube.com/watch?v=w8LTj3jPCeI

h. CIA war =Eugenics drug war fake
https://www.youtube.com/watch?v=0LqDjk8vhyc
i. International Drug Trade, Federal Reserve, CIA and the Bush
Admin: (non specific very challenging broad
based report –) (9m)
https://www.youtube.com/watch?v=y7HBV5jp0Zl
j. Mike Ruppert CIA & Drug Running : The phoney drug war: (16m)
https://www.youtube.com/watch?v=qJkFZ4W4bjg
k. (11m) https://www.youtube.com/watch?v=0LqDjk8vhyc
CIA drug trafficking
https://www.youtube.com/watch?v=2M3I9X3gR2A
m. CIA drug consp (1h46m)
https://www.youtube.com/watch?v=w8LTj3jPCel
n. CIA war =Eugenics drug war fake
https://www.youtube.com/watch?v=0LqDjk8vhyc
o. (146m) https://www.youtube.com/watch?v=FrT-FJAgc0l
p. The Mena Connection, Bush, Clinton and CIA Drug Smuggling
(2h21m)
https://www.youtube.com/watch?v=vTIXRy7ssbl
q. Ron Paul:
http://www.huffingtonpost.com/2011/12/30/ron-paul-conspiracy-
theory-cia-drug- traffickers_n_1176103.html

22. An Intermediate Greek-English Lexicon,
Founded Upon the Second Edition of Liddell and Scott's Greek-
English Lexicon University Press, Oxford, England, 1972
(1st Edition 1889).

Part II CAUSES AND PREVENTION
Part II. 1. FOOD

23. (see also 45 – "Junk Food")
a. The Science of Addictive Food:
http://www.youtube.com/watch?v=4cpdb78pWl4
b. Coke & fizzy drinks reference
c. Why to avoid sodas http://wellnessmama.com/379/reasons-to-
avoid-soda/
d. A video (5m) https://www.youtube.com/watch?v=gDMB0lAgAmw
e. http://nutrition.about.com/od/healthyappetizerssnacks/f/how-
much-sugar-in-cola.htm

24. – Artificial sweeteners, obesity & diabetes: Aspartame®,
aka Nutrasweet®, Aminosweet®, Equal, E951, etc.
a. Technical article by U.S. govt National Library of Medicine
http://www.ncbi.nlm.nih.gov/pmc/articles/PMC2892765/

b. Both sides on CBS News. You decide
http://www.cbsnews.com/news/artificial-sweeteners-could-lead-to-obesity-diabetes/
c. Dr Hyman article on artificial sweeteners sabotaging your diet
http://drhyman.com/blog/2010/06/19/artificial-sweeteners-could-be-sabotaging-your-diet/#close
e. Artificial Sweeteners and Weight Gain
http://www.sciencedaily.com/releases/2008/02/080210183902.htm
f. 200% Obesity increase. Video and article
http://www.huffingtonpost.com/2013/07/11/diet-soda-health-risks_n_3581842.html
g. Artificial sweeteners, obesity and diabetes
http://www.cbc.ca/news/health/artificial-sweeteners-tied-to-obesity-type-2-diabetes-1.1352987
h. Obesity, diabetes and heart attacks
http://www.mensjournal.com/health-fitness/nutrition/the-diet-soda-paradox-20130723
i. Video and article Obesity and other issues
http://articles.mercola.com/sites/articles/archive/2012/12/04/saccharin-aspartame-dangers.aspx

25 Artificial Sweeteners, sodas and cancer

a. Artificial Sweeteners cause cancer in rats at levels approved for humans
http://www.medicalnewstoday.com/releases/34040.php
b. Conflict of interest. U.K. Studies linking cancer and premature births. Independent studies find
Aspartame 'guilty' while studies finding Aspartame 'innocent' linked to vested commercial interest
http://www.dailymail.co.uk/news/article-2290544/Aspartame-Cancer-premature-birth-fears-linked-fizzy-drink-sweetener.html
c. U.S. Sodas and cancer. Dr Rasa Rush and others Uni. Medical Center.** Good advice**
http://www.myfoxchicago.com/story/20939173/diet-soda-dangers-new-study-may-link-aspartame-to-cancer
d. MD Janet Hull PhD Authority on soft drinks, artificial and natural sweeteners.
d1. http://www.janethull.com/askdrhull/category.php?id=5
d2. http://www.sweetpoison.com/aspartame-side-effects.html
e. Aspatame: Genetically mutated bacteria faeces: 24min vid
e1. www.youtube.com/watch?v=q7Ih88NVYmg
e2. http://beforeitsnews.com/health/2013/10/thanks-aspartame-gmo-bacteria-poop-causing-blindness-video-2508976.html

26. Stevia drops

http://en.wikipedia.org/wiki/Stevia
from your health shop, or for Australians/NZers, purchase links:
https://t.cfjump.com/t/22247/871/ & http://tinyurl.com/mholrrc

27. Lead Poisoning
a. http://corrosion-doctors.org/Elements-Toxic/Lead-history.htm
b. the first artificial sweetener
    http://io9.com/5877587/the-first-artificial-sweetener-poisoned-lots-of-romans

28. Lead/fluoride/arsenic comparison
See the charts! http://ffo-olf.org/usefulFluorideUseCharts.html

29. World'stop fluoride researcher **Dr Yiamouyiannis**
http://www.rethinkingcancer.org/resources/magazine-articles/7_9-10/fluoride-the-aging-factor.php

30. Fluoride, mind control
a. http://rense.com/general79/hd3.htm
b. Mind Control, & What every mother should know
    http://www.greaterthings.com/Lexicon/F/Fluoride.htm
c. http://members.iimetro.com.au/~hubbca/fluoride.htm
d. http://forum.prisonplanet.com/index.php?topic=3124.0

31. Physical poisoning and carcinogenisis
(cancer creating effects) of Fluoridea.
a good summary, (USA) Dr Dean Burk Phd:
http://www.whale.to/b/fluoride_q.html
b. brief & most informative (RSA) http://www.cranial.co.za/WATER%20FLUORIDATION.htm
c. Exposure to pregnant women and infants to fluoridated water led to significant reduction in IQ, height, weight & lung capacities of children. Med
d. http://beforeitsnews.com/health/2012/03/flouride-linked-to-brain-damage-and-mind-control-1935159.html
e. comparison of caries in countries that fluoridate water and salt to those that don't.
    http://fluoridealert.org/studies/caries01/
f. JA Yamouyiannis PhD. Cancer Rate Highest in Fluoridated Cities. Reprint 3H/7L, Natl Health Fed Bulletin Monrovia, CA 1975

32 Fluoride, cancer etc: "Poison for the Whole Family"
a. http://naturalsociety.com/top-scientist-fluoride-already-shown-to-cause-10000-cancer-deaths/
b. http://www.homeopathicassociates.com/portfolio-item/fluoride-poison-mueller/
c. "Killing us Softly" Fluoridation, skeletomuscular degeneration and

cancer.
http://www.globalresearch.ca/fluoride-killing-us-softly/5360397
(boys 10-19: http://www.theguardian.com/society/2005/jun/12/
medicineandhealth.genderissues

d. (U.S. Nat. Inst of Health: "The likelihood of fluoride acting as a genetic cause of cancer requires consideration."
http://www.ncbi.nlm.nih.gov/pubmed/11512573)

Videos

d. Dr Dean Burke:Fluoride Causes Cancer (8m)
https://www.youtube.com/watch?v=ClqK7XvfLg0
e. Fluoride, cancer, Science and Politics – Dr Burke: (20m)
http://fluoridealert.org/issues/fluorosis/
f. Fluoride: The Bizarre History: Full Documentary (1h)
https://www.youtube.com/watch?v=0JFLP5k57Y4

33. Your own toothpaste

a. The Best Toothpaste! Free recipe by top holistic dentist! 5 Star ratings by Google and Yelp.
http://besttoothpaste.net/
b. Another resource by Mother Nature Network
http://www.mnn.com/lifestyle/natural-beauty-fashion/stories/3-simple-homemade-toothpaste-recipes
c. Toxic toothpaste,Triclosan, Fluoride & toothpaste recipe:
http://worldtruth.tv/stop-using-these-toxic-supermarket-toothpastes/

Fluoride removal:

d. From water: basil (tulsi) http://naturalsociety.com/tulsi-plant-holy-basil-remove-flouride-water-support-pineal-gland-health/
e. From system: turmeric: http://naturalsociety.com/turmeric-can-save-brain-fluoride-poisoning/
Other 5 ways? http://naturalsociety.com/fluoride-treatment-5-ways-to-detox-fluoride/

34. Meat. Animal conditions

a. Farmageddon (1h26m) https://www.youtube.com/watch?v=5uah8LBUbfc
b. Cowspiracy: the website of an epic movie.

35. genetically mutated, teratogenic animals.

a. http://www.google.co.za/search?biw=1366&bih=643&tbm=isch&q=gm+chicken+kfc&revid=1149821779b.
b. http://www.google.co.za/search?q=gm+chicken&tbm=isch&tbo=u&source=univ&sa=X&ei=PcqJU7_7Hseb0 AXZjYCIDA&sqi=2&ved=0CDIQ7Ak&biw=1366&bih=643
c. Pamela Anderson: Kentucky Fried Cruelty http://link.brightcove.

com/services/player/bcpid2071349516001?bckey=AQ~~,
AAAACofXCIE~,cNM8jhH8p6B3jfJts6Muwg9kUO21LJzh&bct
id=69274988001

36. Most **"free range"** chickens are overcrowded, causing uncharacteristic pecking.
This is the standard "free range chicken farming "solution" Not for sensitive viewers.
http://freefromharm.org/animal-cruelty-investigation/debeaking-video-shows-standard-practice-on-free-range-egg-farms/

37. **A healthy, humane and biointegrated way to raise chickens by Joe Salatin**
https://www.youtube.com/watch?v=zgVFmfibjeE#t=570

38. **Gluten**
a. http://authoritynutrition.com/6-shocking-reasons-why-gluten-is-bad/
b. http://gizmodo.com/why-you-might-want-to-rethink-going-gluten-free-1475646469
c. http://sustainablepulse.com/2014/02/19/roundup-linked-global-boom-celiac-disease-gluten-intolerance/#.VBQeq_mSySo

39 **Fortified foods**
a. http://guardianlv.com/2014/06/research-shows-food-fortified-with-vitamins-and-minerals-can-be-toxic/
b. http://www.theguardian.com/business/2010/nov/23/food-book-extract-felicity-lawrence
c. Nestle admission-no longer accessible

40. **Brown bread – coloured white bread**
a. http://www.youthfitafrica.com/get-fit/nutrition/161-the-truth-about-brown-vs-white-breads-
b. http://www.dailymail.co.uk/health/article-1195904/Is-healthy-brown-loaf-just-white-bread-dyed.html
c. http://www.healthambition.com/white-bread-vs-brown-bread/
d. http://www.cbsnews.com/news/white-bread-in-wheat-breads-clothing/
e. http://www.wikihow.com/Tell-if-Bread-Is-100-Percent-Whole-Wheat

41. **Rodent rather eats box than cereal**
http://www.westonaprice.org/health-topics/dirty-secrets-of-the-food-processing-industry/

42. **Spelt, wonder grain**

a. http://thespeltbakers.ca/what-is-spelt/
b. https://www.natureslegacyforlife.com/faqs/what-is-spelt/
c. also good to eat: http://www.thekitchn.com/good-grains-what-is-spelt-49073

43. Bread storage
a. http://www.livesimplybyannie.com/how-to-properly-store-bread/
b. http://www.wikihow.com/Store-Bread

44. Kinesiological testing: refer to 47 for definition of kinesiology

45. Junk "food" industry (see also 23- "Addictive Food")
a. http://beforeitsnews.com/food-and-farming/2013/03/meat-from-1000-cows-in-a-big-mac-ewwwww-chicken-mcnugets-contain-sillie-putty-no-lie-2451144.html
b. http://authoritynutrition.com/15-health-foods-that-are-really-junk-foods/
c. an understatement. http://healthyeating.sfgate.com/junk-food-affects-children-5985.html
d. The Truth about Your Food: Rob Kenner: https://www.youtube.com/watch?v=2Oq24hITFTY
e. The Truth about Food. Episode 1. (59m) https://www.youtube.com/watch?v=JXZ1dH7tJWw and of course much, much more.....

46. Mac Donalds 1000 animals from 5 countries in one patty
http://tv.greenmedinfo.com/meat-from-1000-cows-in-a-big-mac/

47. Kinesiology
a. Definition. http://medical-dictionary.thefreedictionary.com/applied+kinesiology
b. Official Kinesiology site http://icak.com/

48. Chlorine & Cancer
a. http://www.globalhealingcenter.com/natural-health/chlorine-cancer-and-heart-disease/
b. http://www.stopcancer.com/Water_%20EPA.htm

49. alt public ways of purifying water, **Ultra Violet, Ozone**
a. http://www.newsworks.org/index.php/local/new-jersey/48766-many-municipalities-find-uv-light-a-greener-way-to-purify-water Ozone
b. http://www.comsol.com/blogs/water-purification-using-ozone/
c. http://www.biozone.com/ozone_water_treatment.html

50. Water purification using peroxide and ionic or colloidal silver in airlines, spacecraft & for outdoor enthusiastsa.

a. for aircraft-silver and peroxide.
http://www.skykem.co.uk/elsil-purifier
b. outdoor various water filter/purification systems :
http://www.outdoorgearlab.com/search.php?ftr=water+filters&ogl_search_marker=1

51. **Bottled water,** sunlight, temperature extremes. Dangers of bottled water.
a. Highly technical study by University of Frankfurt:
http://www.plosone.org/article/info%3Adoi%2F10.1371%2Fjournal.pone.0072472
b. Caused Sheryl Crow's breast cancer: they consider it an "urban legend" You decide.
http://urbanlegends.about.com/od/medical/a/bottled-water.htm
c. Online journal http://www.businessinsider.com/bottled-water-is-more-dangerous-than-tap-water-2013-1
d. PBA's, xenestrogens from plastic bottles:
http://health.westchestergov.com/bisphenol-a-and-phthalates

52. **"John" Hopkins University and Dr Fujimoto** on plastics and microwave www.rense.com/general72/newcancer.htm

53. **Reverse osmosis leaches out minerals & acidifies.**
http://www.waterfyi.com/featured/w-h-o-ya-gonna-believe/

54. **Water purifiers**
a. Pureeffect (best quality, value, service) Speak directly to the boss! http://tinyurl.com/m3hx8w4

55. **Chlorine through skin and inhalation**
*ecosmartusa.com (*according to Malwarebytes® this site was attacked when last checked out.(12/'15)

Other resources
a. http://www.wynman.com/chlorine.html
b. U.S.National Library of Health & Medicine – skin absorption
http://www.ncbi.nlm.nih.gov/pmc/articles/PMC1651599/
c. Dr Coldwell,
c1 Video & Script "gas chamber
http://ihelthtube.com/aspx/viewvideo.aspx?v=95947a06f34f340d
c2 Dr Coldwell's Book. "The Only Answer to Cancer."

56. **Agro Chemicals-Country Living**
a. http://www.telegraph.co.uk/earth/agriculture/3458396/Crop-sprays-a-risk-to-health-rules-High-Court.html
b. http://www.toxicsinfo.org/Lawn/Pesticides%20&%20Cancer.htm

many more sites in Google listing

c. http://scholar.google.co.za/scholar?q=cancer+incidence+countrys ide+agricultural+chemicals&hl=en&as_sdt=0&as_vis=1&oi=schol art&sa=X&ei=6R6KU82KCsm8OZyKgegD&ved=0CCcQgQMwAA

57. Agro Chemicals – Systemic Pesticides: poisons don't wash off. The plant/food becomes the poison

a. http://www.panna.org/issues/food-agriculture/pesticides-on-food
b. http://www.motherearthnews.com/nature-and-environment/ systemic-pesticides-zmaz10onzraw.aspx#axzz2yPpbTvvy

58. Less nutritional value commercial food.
The most academically integrous article I could find.

a. http://journeytoforever.org/farm_library/worthington-organic.pdf
b. wine and organics : http://www.winethegreenrevolution.com/knowledge/agriculture/ traditional-agriculture

59. More life in soil than above

a. http://www.ecomythsalliance.org/2010/10/are-there-more-creatures-above-ground-than-below/
b. http://urbanext.illinois.edu/soil/sb_mesg/sb_mesg.htm

60. Kirlian food photos
http://www.fengshuidana.com/2014/01/21/the-dynamic-cellular-energy-of-your-food-your-life/

61. Animals prefer organic:

a. http://www.gmwatch.org/latest-listing/42-2003/4100-chimps-prefer-organic-animals-reject-gm
b. doctors & animals: http://www.sott.net/article/215172-Avoid-Genetically-Modified-Food-Doctors-and-Animals-Alike-Tell-Us
c. http://msgboard.snopes.com/cgi-bin/ultimatebb.cgi?ubb=print_ topic;f=74;t=000908
d. http://freedom-articles.toolsforfreedom.com/gm-food-animals-dont-eat-it/

Effects of GM fed animals (where animals have no choice of other food)

a. Arpad Pusztai PhD (1m) https://www.youtube.com/watch?v=A-6xWsw7uy0
b. (9m) https://www.youtube.com/watch?v=KNjMJIvI3RY
c. (15m) https://www.youtube.com/watch?v=Onw72ShqbP4
d. rats on GM potatatoes 1 (9m) https://www.youtube.com/ watch?v=KNjMJIvI3RY
e. 2 (6m) https://www.youtube.com/watch?v=HcjoL1-Z_E8

f. GM food Cause Tumours And Severe Organ Damage in Rats!
    https://www.youtube.com/watch?v=z55d_bH0450
d. Scientific Studies Prove GMO's Carcinogenic (13m)
    https://www.youtube.com/watch?v=WSJJDc4SYpk
e. GMO Corn & Roundup Cause Cancer Sept 2012-Prof Selarini, Dr
    Anotoniou, ind research org
    http://www.criigen.org: (2m)
f. https://www.youtube.com/watch?v=pDzVBDoXpjE
g. http://sustainablepulse.com/2014/02/19/roundup-linked-global-
    boom-celiac-disease-gluten-intolerance/#.VBQeq_mSySo

Russia reports over 2 million Dead in US As Mysterious Die-Off
Accelerates (GMO CORN).flv (7m)
    https://www.youtube.com/watch?v=7ZYQjaX37nA
    GM food is slow kill mass murder. Nevada Governor 2014 David
    Lory Van Der Beek (37m)
    https://www.youtube.com/watch?v=fWj_t0Qi-Yc

62. GMO's
a. Introduction: http://bestmeal.info/monsanto/facts.shtml
b. U.S. National Library of Medicine, Natural Institute of Health
    admits GM is dangerous
    http://www.ncbi.nlm.nih.gov/pmc/articles/PMC2793308/
c. A brief summary on GMO http://www.youtube.com/
    watch?v=cocp7utUy64&safe=active
d. Seeds of Death (1h20m) & Selection of 200 video clips on You
    Tube
    GMO Watch the video by former GMO proponent Dr Vrain (18m)
    http://www.youtube.com/watch?v=eUd9rRSLY4A&list=PLtsTqO8
    UN5-yNp34CaxyH_IFrbNHrE_U5&safe=active
e. http://www.hoaxorfact.com/Health/russia-suspends-american-
    genetically-modified-corn-over-cancer-fears.html
f. http://www.trueactivist.com/former-pro-gmo-scientist-speaks-out-
    on-the-real-dangers-of-genetically-engineered-food/
g. http://www.relfe.com/2010/pigs_animals_won%27t_eat_gmo_
    corn_food.html
h. F.W.Engdahl
    Open Mind Conference: (1h13m) https://www.youtube.com/
    watch?v=s4qA0Ue_sl4
i   Dr Thierry Vrain: (1h3m) https://www.youtube.com/
    watch?v=l8l4ePHnJbc
j. The World according to Monsanto (1h49m)
k. Seeds of Death-Obama signs
    https://www.youtube.com/watch?v=eUd9rRSLY4A
    https://www.youtube.com/watch?v=2g4LN9xGdng
l. Monsanto Documentary-must watch (1h5m)

https://www.youtube.com/watch?v=omtYlsG1P5U

m. Monsanto, the most Evil Company in the World (102m) (warning – horrific pics!)
https://www.youtube.com/watch?v=UcwmpC9KQzo

Kids speak out against GMO's!
a. **11-year-old boy**
https://www.youtube.com/watch?v=SvVZwJbs54c
b. **Rachel Parent.**
Watch this 14 year old girl "destroy" this old bully! (10m)
https://www.youtube.com/watch?v=Ec1Rvd4lyNw
Alternative (14m)
https://www.youtube.com/watch?v=bvDOYYaZyj4
Rachel on Daytime Toronto (6m)
https://www.youtube.com/watch?v=HheOeHvWAWU
Rachel challenges the Canadian P.M
https://www.youtube.com/watch?v=wdLNIDA8ApY
Rachel started when she was 12
https://www.youtube.com/watch?v=89aMMkyHrVk
Rachel again: "Reveals one of the Best Kept Secrets in the World": video https://www.youtube.com/watch?v=JHQOX8EVNmE

Shorts/trailers
a. GMO foods are toxic. Dr Coldwell: (10m)
https://www.youtube.com/watch?v=ScbbQ2pYd9I
b. GM Poisoning. Concise & Informative:
http://www.responsibletechnology.org/gmo-dangers/65-health-risks/1notes
c. **Monsanto gmo haters of all Natural Life**
https://www.youtube.com/playlist?list=PLvWXCxDQdNvr4WTaPRX5ojfJRcqdCXBVS
d. Understand What GMO's are doing to your body (13m)
https://www.youtube.com/watch?v=H62ScHZkTXw
e. http://www.anh-usa.org/genetically-engineered-food-alters-our-digestive-systems/
f. Study http://www.responsibletechnology.org/gmo-dangers/65-health-risks/2notes.
g. http://earthblognews.wordpress.com/2010/02/17/genetically-modified-food-will-cause-a-global-humanitarian-disaster/
h. Various GM studies, http://earthblognews.wordpress.com/2010/02/17/genetically-modified-food-will-cause-a-global-humanitarian-disaster/

63. Cannibalistic "golden" rice eating
a. http://foodfreedom.wordpress.com/2011/03/11/usda-okays-rice-

modified-with-human-gene-to-be-grown-on-3000-kansas-acres/ scientific article on "golden" Rice
b. http://janetdrscottjanet.hubpages.com/hub/GM-Food-Golden-Rice Blog on "golden rice & gmo".
c. http://www.godlikeproductions.com/forum1/message1429722/pg2
d. http://www.organicconsumers.org/ge/humangene042505.cfm
e. http://www.dailymail.co.uk/news/article-440302/The-rice-human-genes.html
f. http://www.washingtonpost.com/wp-dyn/content/ article/2007/03/01/AR2007030101495.html
g. http://www.surfingtheapocalypse.net/forum/index.php?id=71186

64. Borgen Project
http://www.borgenproject.org

65. Guicciardi.
http://www.storyleak.com/one-week-us-military-spending-wipe-out-world-hunger/

66. GM & patents Video selection
a. http://www.youtube.com/watch?v=4-ouf_ gmA5o&list=PLB37FD73D065F614E
b. Monsanto food wars: (32m) http://www.youtube.com/watch?v=5TTWwOWvPzA
c. Monsanto wants total control, covers up grave GMO dangers… (26m) http://www.youtube.com/ watch?v=cocp7utUy64&safe=active
d. Farmers Be Warned: Monsanto (1h)Documentary-https://www.youtube.com/watch?v=su0om5L4Bhg Look up "Percy Schmeiser"
e. Your breast milk belong to Monsanto! Monsanto patents human breast milk! https://www.youtube.com/watch?v=1SBjxTv6Amg
f. Nestle & Monsanto patent human mother's milk: http:// removingtheshackles.blogspot.com/2013/04/monsanto-nestle-patent-human-breast-milk.html
g. GM cows also to produce human milk: http://wn.com/monsanto_ now_patents_human_breast_milk

67. Monsanto & milk.
a. Fox fires reporters (10m): https://www.youtube.com/ watch?v=dzXY3c7bDLU
b. A more complete report on milk, Monsanto and rBGH. Short video selection http://www.youtube.com/watch?v=axU9ngbTxKw&list=PLD6B069 6E10502158

c. Got Cancer? Milk Poisoning Cover up….(14m)
http://www.youtube.com/watch?v=znFw3uR-MJY
d. Mutant Milk: The World's Most Dangerous Beverage (3m)
http://www.youtube.com/watch?v=h0awf4sinso&list=PLD6B0696
E10502158&index=6
e. You and Your Milk
http://www.youtube.com/watch?v=zwkwhJuZtbw&safe=active
f. Shocking Secrets about Milk. (also Robert Cohen)
http://www.youtube.com/watch?v=hXCs9-Q_Rb8&safe=active
(6m)
g. Why drinking milk is rocket fuel for cancer (11m)
https://www.youtube.com/watch?v=a1dsWjNv3b0
h. Marketing Milk and Disease Dr John McDougall M.D. (43m)
http://www.youtube.com/watch?v=RKu2n4dMMCM
i . The Dangers of Genetically Engineered Milk
http://www.huffingtonpost.com/samuel-s-epstein/the-dangers-of-
geneticall_b_633955.html

68 Legal system & media on gmo
a. USA health site admission: http://www.anh-usa.org/genetically-
engineered-food-alters-our-
digestive-systems/
b. Mons Corps. Companies that use GMO. Boycott them! (9m)
https://www.youtube.com/watch?v=U3hCR_yCvkk
c. Monsanto Evil. (37m)
https://www.youtube.com/watch?v=NIFAgIlmQdk
d. Bill Maher (4m) https://www.youtube.com/watch?v=csSw3fYnICc
e. Berni Sanders (15m)|
https://www.youtube.com/watch?v=tZtiyAPUCkM
f. GMO foods?How to….(14m)
https://www.youtube.com/watch?v=3HYNBY5IKAQ
g. Keiser Report. Monsanto & the Seeds of Evil (25m)
https://www.youtube.com/watch?v=eiK_RF3ioRw
h. Millions Against(10m) Monsanto. Join!
https://www.youtube.com/watch?v=vj-G6VhUynY
i. How to identify GMO-Free food Not looking at labels-
Read the write-up! (7m)
https://www.youtube.com/watch?v=ze-J5qxC0BQ
j. Alex Jones GM Food Dangers (13m)
https://www.youtube.com/watch?v=DWiJPeGtxQ0
k. Alex Jones.The ultimate Secret Exposed. Full Version
https://www.youtube.com/watch?v=WMwXlikoFrM
l. Mike Pollan: Don't eat any food that's advertised
https://www.youtube.com/watch?v=oV6z_ANDvdY

On a positive note

Mike Pollan. Food Rules for Healthy People and Planet
https://www.youtube.com/watch?v=c31cAdYUvT8

69. **GMO** = Decreased agricultural output
http://www.gmeducation.org/faqs/p149408-gm-crops-do-not-increase-yield-potential.html

70. **India**
a. Monsanto Cotton killing soil as well as farmers
https://www.youtube.com/watch?v=eGI8Bhz35EI
b. Monsanto Suicides in India
https://www.youtube.com/watch?v=TEysFa_IMnA
c. Indian Govt files bio piracy Lawsuit against Monsanto (9m)
https://www.youtube.com/watch?v=ryiu5nd3Ih4

   Philipines.
   10 years deception on GM Corn (25m)
   https://www.youtube.com/watch?v=hCuWs8K9-kI

71. **GMO DNA damage reduced by olive oil**
a. http://naturalsociety.com/organic-olive-oil-reduce-dna-damage-soy-gmos/
b. http://www.organicauthority.com/put-it-on-everything-study-finds-olive-oil-benefits-include-protection-from-gmos/

72. **Indian Organic revolution**
a. Punjab: Ex non organic farmer:
http://www.npr.org/templates/
story/story.php?storyId=104708731
b. Tamil Nadu:
http://infochangeindia.org/agenda/agricultural-revival/
tamil-nadu-s-organic-revolution.html
c. facebook page: https://www.facebook.com/indiaorganicrevolution
d. Book: India's Organic Farming Revolution: What It Means for Our Global Food System http://tinyurl.com/o5qmpwg
e. China's organic revolution: http://orgprints.org/14846/1/14846.pdf

73. **South Africa & maize/corn**
a. https://jhaines6.wordpress.com/2012/12/19/people-in-south-africa-die-when-eating-gm-corn-as-a-staple-food-three-times-a-day-thanks-to-a/
b. http://sustainablepulse.com/2012/09/19/criigen-study-links-gm-maize-roundup-premature-death-cancer/#.VBQeq_mSySo

74. **Dr Mouroutis,** https://www.drmouroutis.com

75. **HPV Gardasil;** amongst many: http://truthaboutgardasil.org/

refer to section on vaccines and reference 201

76. Roundup Ready, Glyphosate

a. http://action.responsibletechnology.org/o/6236/t/0/blast Content. jsp? email_blast_KEY=1150514
b. Roundup ready full length food poisoning videos Jeffrey Smith interviews Dr.Stephanie Seneff about Glycophosphate
b1 The Video. (1h05m) http://vimeo.com/65914121
b2 The full article incl. video http://www.foodrenegade.com/link-between-roundup-ready-gmos-disease/
c. Its Worse than we Thought. Dr. Russell Baylock(52m) https://www.youtube.com/watch?v=wA2GhOCtmBE

77. GMO, bad food vs good good guide

a. Australian True food guide: http://www.nongmoproject.org/press/
b. Canadian Greenpeace Guide. http://gmoguide.greenpeace.ca/shoppers_guide.pdf
c. USA GMA awareness group. http://gmo-awareness.com/shopping-list/
d. Mobile. iphone app shopping guide: http://www.nongmoproject.org/find-non-gmo/iphone-app-shopping-guide/

78. Governments and regions opposing gm

http://www.gmo-free-regions.org/gmo-free-regions/bulgaria.html
a. worldwide marches against GMO/Monsanto-ignored by all big media except RT
b. http://rt.com/news/161176-global-march-against-monsanto/

79. Russian Leader against GMO:

a. (Unsubstatniated)
b. http://www.whatdoesitmean.com/index1778.htm
c. http://sustainablepulse.com/2014/03/28/vladimir-putin-russia-must-protect-citizens-gmos/#.U7mqX_mSy4k
d. http://www.globalresearch.ca/moscow-outlaws-monsanto-russia-puts-gmo-genie-back-in-the-bottle/5382971
e. Video version: Russia warns GMO could lead to WW claim(4m) https://www.youtube.com/watch?v=FYp6NidnFNs

80. Public halts Monsanto factory in Argentina until government bribed

a. http://www.infowars.com/activists-halt-monsanto-seed-plant-construction-in-argentina/ (Jan '14)
b. http://revolution-news.com/malvinas-argentina-200-day-blockade-monsanto/ (April'14)

c. http://revolution-news.com/argentina-activists-arrested-brutal-police-repression-monsanto-law-approved/ (June '14)
d. http://thefreethoughtproject.com/protesters-successfully-delay-monsanto-plant-from-opening-in-argentina/

81. Anti GM movements. (a work in progress, till victory!)
a. USA. http://www.nongmoproject.org/press/
b. Australia. http://www.truefood.org.au/takeaction/

82. Omega Oils: US govt , Drs Reiss, Mercola on omega oils
a. (BIOTRUST AFFILIATE BY 24 JAN)
b. http://articles.mercola.com/sites/articles/archive/2011/11/11/everything-you-need-to-know-about-fatty-acids.aspx
c. http://www.globalhealingcenter.com/natural-health/benefits-of-omega-3-6-9-fatty-acids/
d. http://www.webmd.com/drugs/2/drug-149633/fish-oil-omega-3-6-9-oral/details

83 Dr Spiess.
Omega supplement: Rather than sell you supplements, in my opinion it is best to stick with book recommendations: cheaper and as good if not better than anything I can recommend or sell online, unless convincing evidence subsequently emerges to the contrary (update to subscribers and on site).

84. Anti-cancer foods
by Dr Chakravarty.
http://www.hope4cancer.com/information/lemons-and-cancer.html

Part II 2. OXYGEN, ACIDITY, & SUGAR

85. Dr Warburg, concise info:
http://www.glennsiesser.com/2012/12/why-cancer-and-diseases-cant-survive-in-an-alkaline-body-by-nobel-peace-prize-winner/

86. Oxygen levels fall.
http://blogcritics.org/atmospheric-oxygen-levels-fall-as-carbon/

87 Toxic "table salt"
a. http://en.wikipedia.org/wiki/Anticaking_agent
b. Dr Brownstein: http://www.naturalnews.com/026080_salt_sodium_health.html
c. Dr Michelle Kmiec: http://www.onlineholistichealth.com/truth-sea-salt/
d. Salt that Kills, Salt that Heals (37m) https://www.youtube.com/watch?v=O6V1QKx6JLQ

88. Aspartame from excrement of GM bacteria
a. Video (24m) http://www.youtube.com/watch?v=q7Ih88NVYmg
b. http://beforeitsnews.com/health/2013/10/thanks-aspartame-gmo-
c. bacteria-poop-causing-blindness-video-2508976.html (many more)

89. Excessive sodium, fluoride, chlorine, heavy metals, insufficient potassium & magnesium.
Magnesium-Importance & Lack
a. Importance: http://www.sciencebasedmedicine.org/magnesium-the-cure-to-all-disease/
b. Mg deficiency: http://www.greenmedinfo.com/blog/magnesium-deficiency-symptoms-and-diagnosis
Heavy metal Poisoning in food
c. Cans & children: http://www.ncbi.nlm.nih.gov/pubmed/3653455,
d. Canned fish: http://www.ncbi.nlm.nih.gov/pubmed/2376536
e. http://www.sciencedirect.com/science/article/pii/S0308814698000089,
f. http://medical-dictionary.thefreedictionary.com/cadmium+poisoning

90. Melatonin, Health, Hair Loss, Regrowth, Longevity and Cancer.
a. Melatonin on wiki: http://en.wikipedia.org/wiki/Melatonin
b. melatonin cancer prevention & cure http://www.cancer.org/treatment/treatmentsandsideeffects/complementaryandalternativemedicine/pharmacologicalandbiologicaltreatment/melatonin
c. U.S. Library of med. Melatonin for hair loss & possible regrowth. http://www.ncbi.nlm.nih.gov/pmc/articles/PMC3681103/
d. American cancer society on melatonin. www.cancer.org

91. Melatonin: Best Source
The recommended Melatonin supplement:http://tinyurl.com/qgszcrn

92. Hydrogen Peroxide (whilst I don't agree that H2O2 (or anything else) is a cure-all, it is certainly incredible. Together with Colloidal Silver (later referred to) must definitely rank as the two most versatile and most useful health, (as well as most cost efficient) home and garden substances
available. Essential in every home! (but clearly mark and protect

children from H2O2!)
a. Video: (6m) https://www.youtube.com/watch?v=RPxo3z49GTc
b. Article: http://www.foodgrade-hydrogenperoxide.com/id16.html

93. Calcium Deficiency Symptoms
a. http://www.thebestofrawfood.com/calcium-deficiency-symptoms.html
b. http://www.drweil.com/drw/u/ART02814/calcium

94. Dr Coldwell & Dr Wallach on salt
a. Dr Wallach (6m) https://www.youtube.com/watch?v=_9_0gRpt_ok
b. Dr Coldwell good video (7m- salt on 4th m)
    https://www.youtube.com/watch?v=3k3CizAiC9M
* *A free and most effective excellent natural source of calcium is ground eggshell (pre-heat to prevent possible salmonella), and Sprinkle on food or add to banana shakes (which hold it in suspension).*

95. Alkalizing supplement
At the time of writing I do not recommend alkalizing supplements other than the readily available ones proposed in this book, which are just as effective, cheaper and more convenient.

96. Ioniser
email me or refer periodically to cancerfree.cf for- the latest developments and best values in this quickly evolving field.

97. Anti carcinogenic tea and coffee
a. Fred Hutchison research ctr, Harvard:
    http://www.health.harvard.edu/fhg/updates/update0406c.shtml
b. http://fhcrc.org/en/news/spotlight/imports/coffee-nd-tea-consumption-in-ssociation-with-prostate-cncer-r,html
c. http://drweil.com/drw/u/QAA400968/coffee-and-Cancer-Risk.html
d. http://www.rawstory.com/rs/2011/0815/study-explaains-coffee-anti-cncer-effect/
e. http://www.sciencedily.com/releses/2003/10/031015031251.htm
f. http://www.nutraingredients.com/Research/New-step-in-understanding-coffee-s-anti-cancer-action

98. U.S.Library of Medicine on herbs & spices
a. basic.
    http://www.nicbi.nlm.nih.gov/pubmed/18499033
b. more detail.
    http://www.ncbi.nlm.nih.gov/books/NBK92774
c. Biblical Cannabis:(2h15m): www.youtube.com/watch?v=w0bH6Z_OSp8&safe=active

Part III Chapter 3. EMOTIONS

99. Comte St. Germaine Quote:
a. Quote:http://maverickysm.blogspot.com/2011/02/todays-quote.htm
Sites on Comte St. Germaine
b. http://alchemylab.com/count_saint_germain.htm
c. http://revolutionizingawareness.com/documentaries/st-germains-world-trust/

100. Dr Coldwell Quote:
From his book *"The Only Answer to Cancer."* – He recommends a similar approach to this book. http://tinyurl.com/nrx5eb6

101. Laughing out cancer
http://www.healingcancernaturally.com/real-life-healing-stories.html

102. Laughter references massage
a. http://www.peacetreehealing.com/laughter-yoga-usa/health-benefits/
b. Dr Frank Lipman
http://www.drfranklipman.com/comic-relief-the-healing-power-of-laughter/
c. www.cancercenter.com/treatments/laughter-therapy/

103. Water as Prime constituent
a. Water, salt, Diet, Exercise: Dr Batmanghelidj-(2h10m) Most informative on ALL elements on nutrition & Medicine! See it, even if in stages!
https://www.youtube.com/watch?v=8xwezilaUMo

The Memory of Water
a. -*-"The-Miracle-of-Water."-Dr.Masaru-Emoto
A"Must-Read!"–Truth-is-indeed-stranger-than-your-wildest-dreams!
http://tinyurl.com/npo3hvr
b. The memory of water (10m)
https://www.youtube.com/watch?v=BWYIMSHOGBw
c. Water's Memories (49)
https://www.youtube.com/watch?v=59iuelCL0MQ
d. Water has Memory (1h25m)
https://www.youtube.com/watch?v=uNzbiLpnWX8
e. Dr Emoto Water Crystals (35m)
https://www.youtube.com/watch?v=PDW9Lqj8hmc
Comprehensive Playlist Dr Emoto:
f. https://www.youtube.com/playlist?list=PLYq0WlernBA6Q6L3

xd_KKpjl3OocBV05i

g. Water, the Great Mystery video: Science & Religion Converge (1h25m):
https://www.youtube.com/watch?v=FbDJr6M0uPY
If it is taken off youtube for copyright reasons, it can be bought in NTSC (North American format DVD) at:
http://tinyurl.com/lhzxfpm

104. Rice Consciousness Experiment, inspired by Dr Emoto:
https://www.youtube.com/watch?v=31shlv5Z71A

105. Water, basis of homoeopathy
If thoughts can thus affect water, Imagine what it can do to you (20m)
a. https://www.youtube.com/watch?v=FrRD10dLK1o
b. http://www.i-sis.org.uk/WaterRemembers.php
c. Water, a Natural Malleable computer (1h26m)
https://www.youtube.com/watch?v=j51I7YYua_Y
d. http://www.naturalnews.com/029940_homeopathy_scientist.html

106. Cancer Stats
Male and female:
http://www.wcrf.org/cancer_statistics/cancer_frequency.php#BOTH
Male:
http://www.wcrf.org/cancer_statistics/cancer_frequency.php#MEN
Female:
http://www.wcrf.org/cancer_statistics/cancer_frequency.php#WOMEN

107. Mandela on resentment poison
http://www.goodreads.com/quotes/144557-resentment-is-like-drinking-poison-and-then-hoping-it-will

4. ELECTROMAGNETISM

108. William Rea quote:
a: http://www.electromagnetichealth.org/quotes-from-experts/
b: an article on electromagnetism:
http://www.ecolibria.com.au/Resources/electromagnetic-radiation-emr-and-potential-adverse-health-affects
c: advanced but informative:
http://jackkruse.com/emf-5-what-are-the-biologic-effects-of-emf/

109. Cellphone impact on children
http://www.internationalparentingassociation.org/

BrainDevelopment/cellphones.html

110. Cellphone freq military
a. http://www.whale.to/b/rifat.html
   cell phone, microwave & mind control:
b. http://www.cancer.gov/cancertopics/factsheet/Risk/cellphones

111. Cell phones and cancer:
a. The Warnings are in small print: http://consumers4safephones.
   com/apple-warns-customers-to-never-use-or-carry-an-iphone-in-
   your-pocket/
b. Cell phone safety: What the FCC didn't test: http://content.time.
   com/time/magazine/article/0,9171,2029493,00.html
c. Video. Fact: Cellphones cause cancer: Dr Coldwell (4m)
   https://www.youtube.com/watch?v=viJlocZ16j4
d. Dr Sinatra article:
   http://www.drsinatra.com/do-cell-phones-cause-cancer
   http://www.drsinatra.com/cell-phone-radiation-risks/
e. Santosh Kesari:
   https://www.youtube.com/watch?v=MENepGB3GCk
d. CNN: Dr Sanjay Gupta (20m)
   https://www.youtube.com/watch?v=kL2ncKs9K8o
d. Dr Henry Lai-semi technical (16m)
   https://www.youtube.com/watch?v=JrBjQJhHfzk
e. Dr Devra Davis addressing National Institute of Environmental
   Health Sciences (1h2m)
   https://www.youtube.com/watch?v=wNNSztN7wJc
   Dr Martin Blank, and many
f. NEW Urgent warning to all cell phone users:
   http://articles.mercola.com/sites/articles/archive/2012/06/16/emf-
   safety-tips.aspx
g. "Stephen King was Right. Cell Phones can Kill You…. and Your
   Kids" Cati O'Keefe.
   http://www.greenbuildermedia.com/blog/dead-zones-cell-phones-
   can-kill
h. Video. Neurosurgeon Dr. Keith Black & Dr Mercola (6m)
   (radiation protection, refs 113,116/7/8)
   https://www.youtube.com/watch?v=4-95GSTJk78

112. Experimentation-phone radiation
a. https://www.youtube.com/watch?v=e-XW4wOJqjQ
   G4 phones don't pop corn any more
b. thermal images (2m)
   https://www.youtube.com/watch?v=E-RnjkjoJxo
c. plant (5m):
   https://www.youtube.com/watch?v=zmggRlfy4Xg

The TRUTH about CANCER **197**

d. Smart meters/Cell Phones/ Microwve Heath1(14m)
https://www.youtube.com/watch?v=FPbcGK0OeSo

2 (14m) https://www.youtube.com/watch?v=_Qqg2kXgWSc

113 Tubephones for safe cell phone calls, especially for children
http://tinyurl.com/q2k986f

114. Masts, & schools
a. http://altermedicine.org/childhood-leukemia-and-electromagnetic-fields/
b. http://www.radiationresearch.org/10-uncategorised/285-scientific-studies-reveal-that-phone-masts-cause-cancer
c. http://wiredchild.org/component/content/article/46-hidden/77-phone-mast-studies.html
d. http://www.dailymail.co.uk/news/article-449077/Row-cover-mobile-phone-masts-cancer-finding.html
e. http://www.hese-project.org/hese-uk/en/niemr/cellfeedback.php
f. http://www.mast-victims.org/

115. wifi vs ethernet cord
a. http://www.news.com.au/technology/gadgets/new-research-suggests-wifi-signals-could-be-more-harmful-than-we-thought/story-fnjwukfu-1226785092950
b. http://www.pocket-lint.com/news/125892-wi-fi-dangerous-plants-near-routers-are-dying
c. children, wi fi & cell: http://articles.mercola.com/sites/articles/archive/2013/09/21/cell-phone-wifi-radiation.aspx
d. Natural news: http://www.naturalnews.com/041082_wi-fi_wireless_internet_health_effects.html#
e. Scientific studies: http://www.activistpost.com/2013/10/34-scientific-studies-showing-adverse.html

116. Home, Office and other space radiation transmuters
a. Europe based Contact Dr Bindi, AP001 at info@ bioprotectivesystems.com or call her on +441162676599 (U.K-GMT) for comprehensive information for your specific needs.
b. USA based. Paulo Esaamora www.esaamoraa.com. He gives readers a good price.

117. Make your own orgonite:
a. http://www.orgonite.info/how-to-make-orgonite.html
Video (7m):
b. https://www.youtube.com/watch?v=ccS70UQE0fE&safe=active

118. Compact and wearable anti radiation devices

Contact Dr Bindi, AP001 at info@bioprotectivesystems.com or call her on +441162676599 (U.K-GMT) for comprehensive information for your specific needs.

119. CRT child leukaemia:

http://www.altermedicine.org/childhood-leukemia-and-electromagnetic-fields/

120. Online verification found. You may choose to take my word for it.

121. Electric blanket & radiators

a. brain tumours:
http://www.ncbi.nlm.nih.gov/pubmed/8633600
b. breast cancer, American Journal of Epidemliogy:
http://aje.oxfordjournals.org/content/152/1/41.full
c. Dr Weil & Washington University:
http://www.drweil.com/drw/u/QAA400236/Can-Heating-Pads-Cause-Cancer.html
d. Uni. Wisconsin. EMF transmission& Safe Distances:
https://people.uwec.edu/piercech/EMF/

122. Fridge mags: "university danger findings" unfounded.

a. As safe: http://what-cancer.blogspot.com/2012/09/fridge-magnets-is-it-true-that-they.html
b. http://www.hoax-slayer.com/refrigerator-door-magnet-warning.shtml

123. Indoor plants

a. http://www.groomedhome.com/gardening/indoor/8-air-purifying-indoor-plants
b. http://thisgreenearth.wordpress.com/2011/04/07/top-10-plants-to-improve-indoor-air-quality/

124. Cannabis: radiation absorber, Dr Emoto Fukushima:

http://www.naturalcuresnotmedicine.com/category/dr-masaru-emoto

125. Cannabis Anti carcinogen & treatment

http://bigthink.com/devil-in-the-data/marijuana-for-cancer-prevention

126. Plants VOC, NASA, Sick building syndrome

a. http://en.wikipedia.org/wiki/NASA_Clean_Air_Study
b. http://www.diyncrafts.com/4457/home/top-10-nasa-approved-houseplants-improving-indoor-air-quality

c. http://www.mnn.com/health/healthy-spaces/photos/15-houseplants-for-improving-indoor-air-quality/a-breath-of-fresh-air

Sick Building Syndrome
d. http://en.wikipedia.org/wiki/Sick_building_syndrome,
e. http://www.ncbi.nlm.nih.gov/pmc/articles/PMC2796751/
f. http://www.epa.gov/iaq/pdfs/sick_building_factsheet.pdf
g. http://www.nhs.uk/conditions/sick-building-syndrome/Pages/Introduction.aspx
h. http://consumer.healthday.com/encyclopedia/asthma-and-allergies-4/asthma-news-47/sick-building-syndrome-is-your-office-making-you-sick-646729.html

127. Printers must be ventilated:
a. http://www.lhc.org.uk/wp-content/uploads/2012/10/Factsheet-Photocopiers-laser-printers.pdf
b. Xerox instrructions. http://www.xerox.com/downloads/usa/en/e/ehs_ventilation_memo_2002.pdf
c. http://www.healthxchange.com.sg/healthyliving/HealthatWork/Pages/Your-Office-Photocopier-Is-Not-as-Harmless-as-You-Think.aspx

128. Synthetics:
a. http://www.totalhealthmagazine.com/articles/allergies-asthma/consumers-beware-toxins-lurking-in-your-clothing.html
b. http://kriscarr.com/blog/hidden-dangers-of-conventional-fabrics/. Nylon and cystitis: http://health.doctissimo.com/womens-health/about-cystitis/cystitis-myths-debunked.html

129. Fluorescent to L.E.D. lighting
a. comparison: http://www.designrecycleinc.com/led%20comp%20chart.html
b. more info. No affiliation. http://lifx.co/lighting101/advantages/led-vs-fluorescent/
c. google fluorescent vs led lighting

130. Microwave ovens:
Microwave ovens kill food, and eventually You! Dr Coldwell (13m)
a. https://www.youtube.com/watch?v=ScbbQ2pYd9I
b. Barry Trower – Microwaves (14m) https://www.youtube.com/watch?v=z99_SzoXZdY
c. Microwave weaponry use on people (32m): https://www.youtube.com/watch?v=aMMEQNnSZlo
d. Cooking of Humanity (1h32m): www.youtube.com/watch?v=JojdEH0nzos
e. Lecture at Open Mind Conference – 2 parts
e1 (1h.31m) https://www.youtube.com/watch?v=5xgJmeQaQmc

e2 (1h.50m) https://www.youtube.com/watch?v=UhcuSEHVOSM

f. http://foodbabe.com/2012/07/30/why-its-time-to-throw-out-your-microwave/

131 Schoolgirl microwave oven experiments

a. http://preventdisease.com/news/12/041712_Students-Experiment-Shows-How-Microwaved-Water-Kills-Plants-After-Just-Days.shtml

b. http://www.naturalnews.com/031929_microwaved_water_plants.html#
This is another easily duplicable experiment, so why not try it yourself? In order to avoid influencing the experiment by your thoughts, have another person place microwaved and kettle boiled water in two equal containers, labelled 1 & 2, or A & B. You must not know which is the microwaved water for at least two weeks, after which any difference in bean seed germination should be noticed. Use at least three seeds per station to minimise the influence of any variation between individual seeds.

132. "Love" on microwave oven door:
From "The Hidden Messages in Water" by Dr M. Emoto:The in this book will blow you away, and the photographic evidence hard if not impossible to dispute!   http://tinyurl.com/kea2r58

Part II CHAPTER 5. HORMONES

133. Dr Lee's quotes kindly emailed to me by Mr Lee Kroon of Progesterall, www.progesterall.com

134. Charles Huggins, Nobel Laureate
http://www.nobelprize.org/nobel_prizes/medicine/laureates/1966/huggins-bio.html

135. "Hormone Balance Made Simple" Dr J Lee
http://tinyurl.com/molbo5b

136. "What your doctor may not have told you about Pre Menopause." Dr J Lee http://tinyurl.com/lyrmbx4

137."What your doctor may not have told you about Menopause." Dr J Lee http://tinyurl.com/n7rum72

138. "Hormone Balance for Men." Dr J Lee http://tinyurl.com/o234sst

139. Pregnancies and breast feeding:
("parity" means full term) pregnancy

a. http://www.ncbi.nlm.nih.gov/pubmed/18497072

b. http://breastcancer.about.com/od/riskfactorsindetail/a/preg_lower_risk.htm

c. http://www.breastcancercampaign.org/about-breast-cancer/
breast-cancer-risk-factors/pregnancy-and-breast-feeding
d. http://www.breastcancercampaign.org/about-breast-cancer/
breast-cancer-risk-factors/pregnancy-and-breast-feeding
e. http://www.medicalnewstoday.com/articles/264796.php

140. Diapers
a. http://www.smallfootprintfamily.com/dangers-of-disposable-
diapers
b. informative, once you click off annoying popups:
http://kimberlysnyder.net/blog/2012/04/03/the-dangers-of-
diapers-and-why-you-should-be-aware/
c. http://www.thinking-about-cloth-diapers.com/eco-friendly-
diapers.html
d. http://twentysixcats.com/blog/2011/02/11/the-cloth-diaper-
argument/
e. a cloth diaper company answers some questions. I am in no
way affiliated to this particular brand or benefit from it:
http://www.blueberrydiapers.com/Cloth-Diapering-FAQs

141. Feminine hygiene
a. http://www.ncbi.nlm.nih.gov/pmc/articles/PMC3948026/
b. Monsanto is raping you!
http://www.naturalnews.com/051669_tampons_glyphosate_
GMO_cotton.html
c. Reccomended: maxim healthy natural fibre feminine hygeine:
Rebecca at www.maximhy.com
d: Recommended:the best feminine reusable menstrual cup:
http://tinyurl.com/m2j2v9y

142. **"John" Hopkins** on xenestrogens, microwave. Apparently not
from JHU, but good reading nonetheless and reputedly by
Dr Fujimoto, endorsed by Drs Coldwell,Weil, Mercola and other
prominent ex pharma-medical doctors; FDA does not agree.
a. on cancer http://www.oes.org/page2/22819~Cancer_Update_
from_John_Hopkins_Hospital.html
b. plastics in microwave oven http://csn.cancer.org/node/176699
d. discourse on article: http://www.davidsuzuki.org/what-you-can-do/
queen-of-green/faqs/toxics/is-it-safe-to-microwave-plastics/
c. Dr David Suzuki advises on plastics: http://www.davidsuzuki.org/
what-you-can-do/queen-of-green/faqs/toxics/is-it-safe-to-
microwave-plastics/
d. Harvard University vague on the issue, relegating responsibility to
the FDA. Would you?
http://www.health.harvard.edu/fhg/updates/update0706a.shtml

143. "Air fresheners"
a. M Cook.PhD: http://www.care2.com/greenliving/exposed-cancer-causing-toxins-found-in-air-fresheners.html
b. http://www.naturallifemagazine.com/0810/airfresheners.htm
c. http://healthwyze.org/index.php/component/content/article/158-
d. why-air-fresheners-are-a-terrible-health-compromising-idea.html
e. http://healthwyze.org/index.php/component/content/article/184-
f. how-air-fresheners-are-killing-you.html
g. http://foodmatters.tv/articles-1/the-dangers-of-air-fresheners-plus-10-natural-alternatives
DIY Natural, Healthy Air Fresheners
h. http://www.naturallivingideas.com/diy-ideas-to-make-your-home-smell-amazing/
i. http://www.rodalenews.com/natural-air-fresheners
j. http://livinthecrunchylife.blogspot.com/2013/06/diy-baking-soda-air-freshener-jars.html
k. http://naturehacks.com/how-to-make-your-own-natural-air-fresheners/
l. http://www.theprairiehomestead.com/2013/06/homemade-air-fresheners.html
m. Car Air Freshener: http://brownthumbmama.com/2014/10/natural-car-air-freshener.html or buy natural air fresheners

144. Electrical vaporizer: None particularly recommended at time of writing. Work in progress Updates in newsletter & on site.

145. Deodorant: (check updates on cancerfree.cf/resources)
a. odourless men's favourite: http://tinyurl.com/oqu7vkc
b. Truly's for men & women: http://tinyurl.com/p77allr
b. Truly's. http://tinyurl.com/n5pjtnq
c. popular-with-men&athletes-http://tinyurl.com/oqu7vkc

146. Make your own deodorant: some repetition in references but I find that it encourages you to make it.
a. http://wellnessmama.com/1523/natural-deodorant/
b. deo stick. Try various oils, but Tea Tree best antibacterial http://www.wikihow.com/Make-Stick-Deodorant
c. http://www.crunchybetty.com/all-roads-lead-to-the-pits-homemade-deodorant
d. http://www.instructables.com/id/Deodorant/

147. Detergents, soap, cleaners – make your own:
http://www.naturalawakeningsmag.com/Natural-Awakenings/April-2014/Homemade-Eco-Cleaners/

148. oestrogen quiz:
http://www.johnleemd.com/store/resource_hormonetest.html

149. home saliva test
(best test supplier update in newsletter or on http://cancerfree.cf)

150. saliva vs blood test ref:
a. http://womeninbalance.org/choices-in-therapy/hormone-testing/
b. http://www.zrtlab.com/saliva-questions

151. Pregnant mare urine:
a. http://www.peta.org/issues/animals-used-for-experimentation/
   animals-used-experimentation-factsheets/premarin-
   prescription-cruelty/
b. http://www.horsefund.org/pmu-fact-sheet.php
c. http://www.lcanimal.org/index.php/campaigns/other-issues/horses
d. http://www.redrover.org/about-premarin
e. http://dunsgathan.net/horses/pmu.htm
f. similar info with contents of Prematin listed.
   http://www.premarin.org/

152. Progestin not progesterone
a. http://www.huffingtonpost.com/christiane-northrup/hormone-
   therapy-synthetic_b_361570.html
b. Dangerous fraudulent claim by Mayo Clinic, citing progestin (not
   progesterone) as a "female hormone"
   http://www.mayoclinic.org/drugs-supplements/estrogen-
   and-progestin-combination-ovarian-hormone-therapy-oral-route/
   description/drg-20070172

153. ProgestIN worsens cancerous affects of oestrogen, nat prog
doesn't
http://www.ncbi.nlm.nih.gov/pmc/articles/PMC1974841/

154. ProgestERONE Reverses cancerous effects of Oestrogen
a. http://www.thelancet.com/journals/lancet/article/PII0140-
   6736(90)93017-J/fulltext
b. http://www.ion.ac.uk/information/onarchives/breastcancer

155. Natural progesterone purchase link
http://tinyurl.com/m32v7yk
156. Dr Lee & Lancetosteoporosis reference:
http://www.thelancet.com/journals/lancet/article/PII0140-
6736(90)93017-J/fulltext

157. Breast Cancer Prevention:
Nutritionalist: Nat prog balances oestr

http://www.ion.ac.uk/information/onarchives/breastcancer

158. Recommended cream for men and women:
get bioidentical/natural progesterone here
with highest progesterone concentration,(4% vs 1,5% std)
no artificial or harmful ingredients and competitive pricing
http://tinyurl.com/m32v7yk

159: Fish – rivers and oceans
a. poisoned river, fish: http://www.theguardian.com/
b. environment/2012/jun/02/water-system-toxic-contraceptive-pill

160. Osteoporosis, cancer, etc and hormones
a. "Every Woman Should Read This Chapter Now"
    http://www.thedoctorwithin.com/women/every-woman-needs-to-
    read-this-chapter-now/
b. Dr Lee Interview:
    http://www.yourlifesource.com/dr-john-lee-interview.htm

161. Oestradiol female lubricant
a. Product website/ 1st line:"Estrogens increase the chance of getting
    cancer of the uterus" :
    http://www.estracecream.com/
b. http://www.drugs.com/mtm/estrace-vaginal-cream-topical.html
c. http://www.drugs.com/pro/estrace-cream.html
d. http://www.rxlist.com/estrace-vaginal-cream-side-effects-drug-
    center.htm
e. http://www.everydayhealth.com/drugs/estrace-vaginal-cream

162. Natural birth control
Counting days between periods can be unreliable, especially
if your periods are irregular or if you are having emotional issues.
Temperature and learning about vaginal mucus thickness is much
more reliable, but remember that not even this is totally "safe" if
one takes into account a three day lifespan of sperm in a woman;
in fact fertility timing kits are recommended more for ensuring
conception than contraception, as sperm lives for up to 5 days in
a woman's body,long before a woman shows signs of ovulation;
also remember that both women and men (through a woman's
pheromones) are more amorous during fertile times! (which is
why the traditional "Catholic NFA – "Natural Fertility Awareness" is
such a failure; it is so easy/tempting to 'conveniently' lose count)
a. http://articles.mercola.com/sites/articles/archive/2010/07/10/real-
    contraceptive-choices-alternatives-to-risky-hormone-pills-
    patches-and-shots.aspx
b. http://www.greenideareviews.com/2012/06/17/all-natural-birth-

control-symptothermal-fertility-awareness-natural-family-planning-review-does-it-work/

c. The "mucus" method:
http://nfp.marquette.edu/nfp_quick_inst_mucus.php
(use physical barriers on "high fertility" days) Note: No contraception/fertility method has ever been or claimed to be "100% safe".

c. Not ratified**** http://www.nfmcontraception.com/*****

d. Not ratified beyondfertility.net

163. Buyer's guides
a. http://www.nongmoshoppingguide.com/
b. http://www.choice.com.au/reviews-and-tests/food-and-health/food-and-drink/organic-and-free-range/organic-food.aspx
c. http://www.helpguide.org/articles/healthy-eating/organic-foods.htm

164. Frequent (good) sex good:
a. http://www.cnn.com/2010/HEALTH/01/07/sex.health.benefits/
b. http://www.webmd.com/sex-relationships/guide/sex-and-health
c. men's health:
http://www.menshealth.com/sex-md/sex-health-benefits

Part II 7. THE PHYSICAL BODY

165. Swami Vivekananda
a. http://en.wikipedia.org/wiki/Swami_Vivekananda
b. http://thinkexist.com/quotation/the_moment_i_have_realized_god_sitting_in_the/342386.html
c. http://www.brainyquote.com/quotes/authors/s/swami_vivekananda.html
d. http://prevalux.com/teachings-of-swami-vivekananda-5b7ac-free-5617a

166. Sun screens. A Must Watch: (2.34m)
https://www.youtube.com/watch?v=5Rym0Zcdl5c
b. Dr Elizabeth Lourdes: (3m)
https://www.youtube.com/watch?v=fGG-84e1kaw
c. Dr Ann Louise: Sunscreen: Shocking Research Exposed
c1: Part 1 (11m) https://www.youtube.com/watch?v=ZpQdNA2XplQ
c2: Part 2 (11m) https://www.youtube.com/watch?v=UAEdpjmYu3A
c3: Part 3 (13m) https://www.youtube.com/watch?v=t4CrmeTef1w

167. Recommended Natural sun screens. No dangerous ingredients.

a   http://tinyurl.com/m32v7yk

168. Home made sun screens nice full article http://beforeitsnews.com/alternative/2014/07/why-you-need-to-make-your-own-sunscreen-2987698.html

169. Sun info, ebook and video

a.   US National Library of Medicine:
http://www.ncbi.nlm.nih.gov/pubmed/18550652

b.   American Society for Clinical Nutrition: http://ajcn.nutrition.org/content/80/6/1678S.full

c.   book: http://www.naturalnews.com/specialreports/sunlight.pdf

d.   video: http://tv.naturalnews.com/v.asp?v=5A62FC73922FD51A88E62E42C5A0AD5E

170. Dangers in (commercial) cosmetics

a.   http://www.ewg.org/research/exposing-cosmetics-cover/true-horror-stories-of-cosmetic-dangers

b.   http://www.dailymail.co.uk/health/article-108549/Danger-hides-make-up.html

c.   http://www.ewg.org/research/exposing-cosmetics-cover/true-horror-stories-of-cosmetic-dangers

d.   http://www.cncahealth.com/explore/learn/green-living/the-real-cost-of-beauty-dangerous-toxins-lurking-in-your-cosmetics

e.   Dr Warns of Dangerous Chemicals in Cosmetics- +video: http://fox4kc.com/2014/11/06/doctor-warns-of-dangerous-chemicals-found-in-popular-cosmetics/

f.   Major Risks from Cosmetic and Personal Care Products: http://www.drfranklipman.com/risks-from-toxic-ingredients-in-cosmetics-personal-care-products/

g.   The Truth -slideshow: http://www.webmd.com/beauty/makeup/ss/slideshow-truth-about-beauty-product-dangers

171. Recommended Safe Cosmetics Americas

a.   Sodashi: "world's #1 Skincare": http://tinyurl.com/q7538t8

172 Recommended Safe Cosmetics, rest of world

a.   World. Sodash "world's#1 skincare" select region, top right of site: https://t.cfjump.com/t/22247/10533/http://tinyurl.com/q7538t8

b.   Europemany to be found all over Europe

c.   Australia & NZ
Full range of top skin care and 100% natural cosmetics: http://tinyurl.com/op5g7bu

Other approved products & Countries: Updates on site and with newsletters

173. Refs173, 174 – Extensive list. Refer to site

174. Refs173, 174 – Extensive list. Refer to site

175. Homemade natural deodorants see 146

176. Bras make breasts sag: latest findings.
http://www.medicalnewstoday.com/articles/259073.php

177. No bra reduces likelihood of breast cancer
a. http://www.brafree.org/
b. http://all-natural.com/bras.html
c. http://articles.mercola.com/sites/articles/archive/2009/05/19/Can-Wearing-Your-Bra-Cause-Cancer.aspx

178. What your doctor may not tell you about breast cancer.
Dr Lee book
http://tinyurl.com/m8u69bx, or http://tinyurl.com/lf4t9go

179. Prostate massage
http://www.prostate-massage-and-health.com
180. prostate wand: & for top-notch prostate support products:
http://zfer.us/Z9745
181. Kegel exercises (for full pubic health not just incontenance!)
a.men: http://www.webmd.com/urinary-incontinence-oab/kegel-exercises treating male urinary incontinence
video:- https://www.youtube.com
watch?v=6xIOveII80A&safe=active
b.women: – http://www.webmd.com/women/tc/kegel-exercises-topic-overview
videos-https://www.youtube.com/
watch?v=wRKhtfbJHdo&safe=active
(and-other-videos-by-Michelle-Kenway)

182. Hormone Balance for Men and Women
a. Men: "Hormone Balance for Men" Dr J. Lee
http://www.amazon.com/dp/ B009274R38/?tag=cancerfree
b. Women: "Hormone-balance-Made-Simple" – Dr J. Lee
http://www.amazon.com/dp/ 044669438X /?tag=cancerfree

183. Couples intimate massage course
Due to demand, this workshop is now available not only to couples, but therapists, singles and even small groups. Book well in advance! Contact on site http://cancerfree.cf

184. Top-Louise Hay books-&Products
a. Meditations-to-Heal-Your-Life http://www.amazon.com/dp/ 1561706892 /?tag=cancerfree

b. Gratitude,a-Way-of-Life- http://www.amazon.com/dp/1561703095/?tag=cancerfree
c. Love-Yourself,-Heal-Your-Life-(WORKBOOK) http://www.amazon.com/dp/0937611697/?tag=cancerfree
d. Power-Thought-Cards-(a-popular-gift) http://www.amazon.com/dp/1561706124/?tag=cancerfree
e. Wisdom-Cards(women's-favourite) http://www.amazon.com/dp/1561707309/?tag=cancerfree
f. Her-#1Best-Seller-You-Can-Heal-Your-Life http://www.amazon.com/dp/1561706124/?tag=cancerfree
g. Heal-your-Life-Companion-Book http://www.amazon.com/dp/ B005LB7AEC/?tag=cancerfree

7. ACIDITY AND FUNGUS

185. Tulio Simoncini videos
Pt 1 of 2 (10m) https://www.youtube.com/watch?v=s0jviLGXRwI
Pt 2 of 2 (10m) https://www.youtube.com/watch?v=OnrxN4N5KCk

186. Transcend cancer (c), for consultation, seminar & to preorder book email on site. http://cancerfree.cf

187. Candida home test
Look out for updates on site

188. Candida quiz:
http://www.nationalcandidacenter.com/candida-self-exams/

189. Acidophilus
a. DIY Acidophilus: http://homestead-and-survival.com/how-to-make-lactobacillus-acidophilus/
b. Buy Acidophilus from the most reputble source: a: http://tinyurl.com/krmytzy
c. http://findyourbalancehealth.com/2013/12/wildfermentedfruitykvass/
d. Home made probiotics: look up "home made probiotics" on youtube

190. Best Candida cure.
a. Highly recommended! Could literally be a life saver!
http://tinyurl.com/lzuyq3j

190.e- Stevia and safe natural sweeteners –
Australia & NZ http://tinyurl.com/mholrrc
Elsewhere, your local health shop is best.

191 Greek Yoghurt

a. health.usnews.com/health-news/blogs/eat-run/2014/05/05/the-health-benefits-of-greek-yogurt
b. http://www.fitday.com/fitness-articles/nutrition/healthy-eating/5-reasons-why-greek-yogurt-is-the-perfect-healthy-snack.html#b
c. 8 Ways Greek Yoghurt Benefits your Health: http://www.healthline.com/health/food-nutrition/greek-yogurt-benefits
d. http://healthyeating.sfgate.com/benefits-greek-yogurt-vs-regular-yogurt-6187.html
e. My Big Fat Greek Yoghurt: Why its Super: http://greatist.com/health/superfood-greek-yogurt
f. http://www.healthyeating.org/Milk-Dairy/Nutrients-in-Milk-Cheese-Yogurt/Yogurt-Nutrition.aspx

8. MEDICINE & ANTIBIOTICS

192. Dr Josh Axe Quote
a. http://draxe.com/conventional-medicine-is-the-leading-cause-of-death/

193. Death by Medicine:
READ THIS and see the video By teams of medical experts:
a. *A Must Read* **Death by Medicine**:. http://www.webdc.com/pdfs/deathbymedicine.pdf
b. *A Must See* Peter Gotzche of Cochrane Collaboration. **"Deadly Medicines & Organised Crime"** (16m)
https://www.youtube.com/watch?v=VIIQVII7DYY#t=43

194. Dr Coldwell. quote a:
a. http://holisticcancerresearch.com/dr-coldwell-all-cancer-can-be-cured-in-less-than-12-weeks.html quote b: video :
b. https://www.youtube.com/watch?v=DgbdNNfotwM (6m20s into 7m video)

195. The Hidden History of Medicine: Mike Adams
http://www.naturalnews.com/specialreports/25-Amazing-and-Disturbing-facts-about-the-Hidden-History-of-Medicine.pdf

196. Psyche-delics= Soul/psyche delic/revealing substances
There are many resources on this, requiring openminded, honest research
a. http://www.breakingopenthehead.com/what_are_psychedelics.htm review or buy the book here: http://tinyurl.com/lmt68gg
b. http://www.salon.com/2014/04/15/6_facts_about_psychedelic_drugs_that_will_totally_blow_your_mind_partner/
c. Aldous Huxley: The doors of Perception
review or buy the book here http://tinyurl.com/nrw582l

d. Terence McKenna: Food of the Gods
   review or buy the book here: http://tinyurl.com/ko5dv9g
e. Don Jose Campos: The Shaman & Ayahuasca: Journeys to Sacred Realms
   review or buy the book here: http://tinyurl.com/ko5dv9g

Videos: Look up "psychedelics and consciousness" on youtube.

197. No such thing as ADHD
a. Bauchmann
   http://www.cchrint.org/2011/05/21/is-adhd-a-fictional-disease/
b. Richard Saul:
   http://www.dailymail.co.uk/health/article-2534632/ADHD-doesnt-exist-Neurologist-claims-condition-masking-problems-causing-needless-use-addictive-drugs.html

198. Ritalin, Psychotropic Drugs and Children.
a. Making a Killing. The Untold Story of Psychotropic Drugging
   https://www.youtube.com/watch?v=Lo0iWh53Pjs (1h34m)
b1. The Drugging of our Children (1h43m)
   https://www.youtube.com/watch?v=26e5PqrCePk
b2. 0-5 years!!!
   https://www.youtube.com/watch?v=gywCn1T-Jug
c1. Ritalin package insert. (Pdf)
   https://www.pharma.us.novartis.com/product/pi/pdf/ritalin_ritalin-sr.pdf
c2. Strattera, another ADD drug package insert. (Pdf)
   http://pi.lilly.com/us/strattera-pi.pdf
d1. Ritalin & Suicide: By no means an isolated case:
   http://www.ritalindeath.com/
d2. Strattera & Suicide:
   http://ritalindeath.com/Strattera-Suicide.htm
e. http://www.dailymail.co.uk/health/article-2002856/Harry-Hucknall-10-killed-taking-Ritalin.html
f. Ritalin & Cancer:
   http://www.preventcancer.com/patients/children/ritalin.htm
g. Ritalin & Legal response:
   http://www.yourlawyer.com/topics/overview/ritalin

199. Big pharma bribes:
Doctors bribed to use adult meds on children:
a. http://www.theguardian.com/business/2012/jul/03/glaxosmithkline-fined-bribing-doctors-pharmaceuticals
b. http://www.thefix.com/content/jj-sued-illegal-promotion-drugs-kids?page=all
c. http://www.abclawcenters.com/blog/2011/04/14/how-drug-companies-bribe-doctors-54446GlaxoSmithKline: GUILTY in

Largest Health Fraud Settlement in US History
d. http://articles.mercola.com/sites/articles/archive/2012/07/16/glaxosmithkline-plead-guilty.aspx
e. China: Pharma CEO pleads Guilty: Doctors bribed with money & sex
http://www.theguardian.com/business/2014/sep/19/glaxosmithkline-china-mark-reilly-deported-uk-guilty-bribery-hunan
f. GlaxoSmithKiline in Poland:
http://www.swadeshionline.in/news/glaxo-smith-kline-bribed-doctors-boost-sales-whistleblower-says

200. Underage Ritalin, forced 'treatment', 'wards of state'
Please send your loving wishes and prayers to these victims of state/medical violence, kidnapping, torture and ieven murder.

Cassandra-Forced Chemo
a. http://wtnh.com/2015/01/10/teen-opens-up-about-forced-chemotherapy-death/
b. http://www.greenmedinfo.com/blog/forcing-chemo-17-year-old-deadly-research-reveals
c. News Video. See how stupid reporters contradict themselves by saying that Caassandra is a minor and cannot take a decision whilst saying that she is "probably influenced by her mother". As for their "statistics" of the "healing potential of chemo"; these are totally false and contradict even the official U.S. govt health stats as referenced in this book.http://www.cbsnews.com/videos/connecticut-teen-with-cancer-breaks-silence-over-forced-chemotherapy/
d. http://www.collective-evolution.com/2015/01/10/17-year-old-forced-against-her-mothers-will-to-undergo-chemotherapy/
e. http://www.courant.com/news/connecticut/hc-teen-battles-chemo-order-0103-20150102-story.html#page=1
f. http://www.courant.com/opinion/op-ed/hc-op-cassandra-my-body-my-life-0109-20150108-story.html
g. Support her facebook page:
"Desperate help to connect with Jackie Fortin
Teen Cassandra Fortin's mom!"
Medical Kidnapping in 50 US States
a. http://medicalkidnap.com/
b. http://healthimpactnews.com/2014/a-history-of-medical-kidnapping-at-phoenix-childrens-hospital/

The above are just the "tip of the iceberg" of children forced to take vaccines, Ritalin®, chemo, etc and kidnapped when parents object. Stand up in supporting these children and families. Your child could be next!

201. Vaccines never saved us from anything.
a. http://healthimpactnews.com/2013/history-and-science-show-vaccines-do-not-prevent-disease/
b. Dr Lorraine Day:
http://www.whale.to/a/day5.html
c. Curtis Cost:
http://www.whale.to/vaccine/cost_i.html
d. Site dedicated to vaccines:
http://thinktwice.com/
e. http://healthimpactnews.com/2013/history-and-science-show-vaccines-do-not-prevent-disease/
f. Polio vaccine:
http://healthimpactnews.com/2013/the-real-history-behind-the-polio-vaccine/
g. History & Sciences how that vaccines do not prevent disease:
http://next-level-nutrition.com/?p=13028
h. http://www.greenmedinfo.com/blog/2013-measles-outbreak-failing-vaccine-not-failure-vaccinate1

202. Toxic content of vaccines, heavy metals, etc
a. **JUST RELEASED. MUST SEE!**
http://www.naturalnews.com/053022_robot_doctors_future_of_medicine_totalitarian_compliance.html
b. 2500x above EPA Limit!
http://www.naturalnews.com/045418_flu_shots_influenza_vaccines_mercury.html
c. Joining the dots…
http://www.sott.net/article/263203-Connecting-the-Dots-Vaccines-heavy-metals-GMOs-and-brain-damage.
d. see "general" reports and videos (208)

203. Autism, sterility, death
a. 100-year-old warning about vaccines by Mahatma Ghandi!
http://www.greenmedinfo.com/blog/gandhis-anti-vaccine-views-ring-true-century-later.
b. Don't vaccinate, by chemist:
http://thepeopleschemist.com/reasons-dont-vaccinate-children-vaccine-supporters-shouldnt-give/
c. Expert paediatrician discusses vaccines 1/11 (10m)
https://www.youtube.com/watch?v=K2lgLj2lf44c.
d. http://www.dailymail.co.uk/news/article-2720333/Did-HPV-vaccine-kill-daughter-Mother-demands-answers-healthy-active-daughter-12-collapses-dies-getting-vaccine.html
e. Measles: Rash of Misinformation:
http://www.greenmedinfo.com/blog/measles-rash-misinformation1
f. Vaccine Cancer, Viruses…. cause all diseases… Dr Rebecca Carley

https://www.youtube.com/watch?v=_vdiorTZvKg (4h44m) ***

204. Vaccine with HIV: (3m)
AIDS in vaccine, and sold knowingly. (Profit in genocide) NBC News.
a. https://www.youtube.com/watch?v=Wf2u7j9FeVI&list=PL3355066 494E284C7
b. http://www.youtube.com/watch?v=wg-52mHIjhs.
Admitted to creating aids Dr Gallo: "peacetime biological warfare"
c. https://www.youtube.com/watch?v=HgiMqgjS-zM

205. Vaccine Population control: (see also 207)
a. HPV vaccination used as population control? Dr Coldwell (7m)
https://www.youtube.com/watch?v=Z__mqgbWwE8
b. 75% kill rate on Mexican children:
http://www.naturalnews.com/049669_vaccine_injury_ depopulation_agenda_deadly_side_effects.html

206. Vaccine Mind control:
a. http://www.drinkyourmulti.com/articles-on-nutrition/vaccination-and-the-mind
b. Dr Russell Blaylock. How Vaccines can harm child brain development (1h28m)
https://www.youtube.com/watch?v=G2e6oGvxDuw

207. Gardasil (HPV vaccine) (see also 205)
Gardasil: HPV Vaccine:
a. http://truthaboutgardasil.org/about-2/
b. The Dangers of the HPV Vaccines Gardasil & Ceravix (17m)
https://www.youtube.com/watch?v=WCA5haGU6sI
c. Young Girls Convulse on Floor after HPV Shot
https://www.youtube.com/watch?v=MvAOoDtbdVI

208. "Small" selection of articles and videos of many.
On Children
a. Expert paediatrician discusses vaccines 1/11 (10m)
https://www.youtube.com/watch?v=K2IgLj2If44
b1. Dr Russell Blaylock. How Vaccines can harm child brain development (1h28m)
https://www.youtube.com/watch?v=7QBcMYqlaDs
b2. Vaccine Truth & Immunotoxicity
https://www.youtube.com/watch?v=JjVR12DZ2oI&list=PLPS7fol eF_i20of66kKOEIrq8LA-pwseF
c. http://childhealthsafety.wordpress.com/graphs/
Can we continue to justify injecting aluminium into children?:
http://www.greenmedinfo.com/blog/can-we-continue-justify-injecting-aluminum-children

d. Dr Mercola. Heavy Metals, glyphosate... children
http://articles.mercola.com/sites/articles/archive/2014/05/08/
heavy-metals-glyphosate-health-effects.aspx

General Articles
e. Healthy Foods, Not Vaccines Dr Mercola
http://articles.mercola.com/sites/articles/archive/2012/08/06/
healthy-foods-not-vaccines.aspx

General Videos
f. Debate on vaccines: Vaccine developers. Heroes or Villains?
Presented by Dr Sherry Tenpenny. (1.6)
https://www.youtube.com/watch?v=DoSHVolyy_4&list=PLPS7fol
eF_i20of66kKOEIrq8LA-pwseF
g. Vaccine Truth & Immunoexcitotoxicity
https://www.youtube.com/playlist?list=PLPS7foleF_
i20of66kKOEIrq8LA-pwseF
h. Dr Wakefield. Vaccine Dis-info
https://www.youtube.com/watch?v=Ft6LwI2ISQw
i. The Untold Story of Vaccines (1h47m)
https://www.youtube.com/watch?v=K1m3TjokVU4
j. (1h47m) Open Mind Conference.
https://www.youtube.com/watch?v=dCDbup1eo8Q
k. Injected. The Truth about Vaccines. (Full panel of specialists)
(2h4m)
https://www.youtube.com/watch?v=_VDzTHONu5g
l. Dr Tenpenny, What the CDC Documents say about Vaccines
https://www.youtube.com/watch?v=M1VwVBmx0Ng
m. Drs SuzanneHumphries and Sherry Tenpenny Vaccines-Get the
Whole Story (54m)
https://www.youtube.com/watch?v=ljlq1wwj7Po
n. Dr R Carley.Vaccines & the Medical Mafia & Others
Pt1-(1h22) Pt2 (1h.26) & more
https://www.youtube.com/watch?v=9WoMps4Pmpo&list=PLMXVn
okDhogs4lu59JWwje35nNsx8clWD
o. ***Vaccines. The silent epidemic....: Gary Null (1h48m)
https://www.youtube.com/watch?v=lJGyN3gCsBg or
https://www.youtube.com/watch?v=K1m3TjokVU4
Autism: Made in the USA (& other videos by G Null)
https://www.youtube.com/watch?v=fwuyxyBUmwY (1h41m)x
p. Shots in the /Dark. Silence on vaccine (1h30)
https://www.youtube.com/watch?v=pnxAsrAK2hw
q. Vaccines. A Complete Fraud (1.08)
https://www.youtube.com/watch?v=kRNFoHOsaw0
r. Dr W. Spencer et al. The vaccine & flu epidemic fraud (1h38m)
https://www.youtube.com/watch?v=sA9adgq5aBc
s. "100 Dead" Vaccine Epidemic

https://www.youtube.com/watch?v=gEq95DyPMjI
t. Silent Epidemic. The Untold Story… (1h48m)
https://www.youtube.com/watch?v=K1m3TjokVU4
u. Shots in the Dark: Silence on Vaccine (1h30m)
http://www.youtube.com/watch?v=pnxAsrAK2hw
v. Lethal Injection: The Story of Vaccination *Scientific explanation*
(2h32m)   https://www.youtube.com/watch?v=7hITYIT02rA

209. GM vaccines:
a. American Law Journal: Dollars for Doctors (29m)
https://www.youtube.com/watch?v=ISwN7-mPo7c
b. Glaxo Klein bribery & corruption(1h7m)
https://www.youtube.com/watch?v=y_RJ9QPG70U
c. Big Pharma's Massive Bribery Network (55m)
https://www.youtube.com/watch?v=dEbWrNL4_SY
J&J
d. Former big pharma whistle blower Gwen Olsen (21m)
https://www.youtube.com/watch?v=zWNLH6hUL2o
d. Dr Viparen: big pharma whistleblower (10m)
https://www.youtube.com/watch?v=Qmi3ihrUHJU
e. Inside pharma ind (22m)
https://www.youtube.com/watch?v=PtalhShZzOY
f. War on health (2h05m) – A "Must see"
https://www.youtube.com/watch?v=ziCTNkV3FBI
https://www.youtube.com/watch?v=AanB_fPq8eU or
(1h38m) https://www.youtube.com/watch?v=h0CQrL5nzwo or
(57m)   https://www.youtube.com/watch?v=tvsjxzkPPZg

ALL THAT GLITTERS....
210. Colloidal Silver-AIDS
This Video by Dr Bob Beck AIDS, Cancer, etc (1h57m)
https://www.youtube.com/watch?v=exMxfj0oCQ8

211. Colloidal Silver Treating Cancer
a. U.S. Govt Health site: Antitumor activity of Coll. Silver:
http://www.ncbi.nlm.nih.gov/pmc/articles/PMC2996348/
b. This Video by Dr Bob Beck will blow your mind! (ref210) (1h57m)
https://www.youtube.com/watch?v=exMxfj0oCQ8
part of Dr Beck's C.S . Cancer treatment protocol: http://www.
cancertutor.com/bobbeck-cs/
c. Independent Cancer Research Foundation: C.S. Protocol for
Cancer: http://www.new-cancer-treatments.org/Cancer/DMSO_
CS.html
d. Alliance for Natural Health: http://www.anh-usa.org/oldest-
antibiotic-shows-promise-as-anti-cancer/
e. http://www.dailymail.co.uk/health/article-2095610/Silver-bullet-
cancer-Metal-kill-tumours-better-chemotherapy-fewer-effects.html

f. C.S. Wonder Miracle for Cancer: http:// undergroundhealthreporter.com/colloidal-silver-a-wonderful-miracle-for-cancer/#axzz3V3LV91P8

g. Breat Cancer. http://greenhealthmatters.com/breast-cancer-treatment-alternatives/

212. Colloidal silver
author's incredible experiences to be posted in newsletters.

213 Buy colloidal silver
I could sell you a lot of colloidal silver, but recommend you buy your own generator to save a lot of money and always have sufficient colloidal silver whenever needed.

214 101 Uses of Colloidal Silver
on cancerfree.cf /cs

215. Buy machine (silver lung)
a. Not cheap but the best: inhaler optional: http://tinyurl.com/opowa4v

b. Whilst I recommend above model, am conducting ongoing research on satisfactory more economical models for suitable particle size and concentration and value for money.
You will be updated in newsletter and site.

Part III CLOSING OUR CASE

216. Dr Watson quote "a Pile of shit"
a. The failed war on Cancer: Informative pdf:
http://www.peopleagainstcancer.com/pdfs/news/20080916n2.pdf

b. What the Cancer Industry Doesn't want you to Know (19m)
https://www.youtube.com/watch?v=7YFS5qlAzgc

c. The Medical Mafia Attack on Alternative Cancer Treatment (1h48m)
https://www.youtube.com/watch?v=DMGWV9mI508

d. The Cancer Conspiracy (1h33m)
https://www.youtube.com/watch?v=Tx7W662gd8M

Part III 1. A CURE TO DIE FOR

217. Dr Hamer quote "a Monument in Hell":
easy read pictorial pdf:(a), related links (b)

a. http://www.germannewmedicine.ca/documents/Chemo%20Intro-e.pdf

b. http://www.whale.to/cancer/cancers1.html

218. Cytochrome P450:
http://www.sciencedirect.com/science/article/pii/
S0027510798000372)

219. Dr Alan Levin M.D. book "The Healing of Cancer"
Book out of print, but various references by Dr Levin at
a. chemo, major cause of cancer" :
http://www.hangthebankers.com/study-chemotherapy-
actually-increases-cancer-growth/   and a similar article:
a1 http://www.indybay.org/newsitems/2013/10/28/18745548.php
b. Death by Doctoring:
http://www.cancertutor.com/deathbydoctoring1/
c. http://www.cureyourowncancer.org/chemo-kills.html

220. Royal North Shore Hospital Cli Oncol
a RColl Radiol) 2005 Jun;17(4):294
b. http://www.ncbi.nlm.nih.gov/pubmed/15630849
c. https://www.burtongoldberg.com/home/burtongoldberg/
contribution-of-chemotherapy-to-five-year-survival-rate-morgan.
pdf

221. U.S. National Institute of Health site:
contributor of cytotoxic therapy U.S. National Libr of med
http://www.ncbi.nlm.nih.gov/pubmed/15630849

222. Arthur Reed book. www.arthurreed.co.za

223. Dr Simoncini website 75% opposed:
a. http://simoncini-cancer-center.com/old_treatments
b. http://www.curenaturalicancro.com/en/75-percent-of-the-
physicians-refuses-chemotherapy-themselves/
c. **Dr Farley: Over 90% oncologists prescribe but refuse**
https://www.ihealthtube.com/video/these-doctors-use-these-
toxins-you-not-their-own-family-members
d. http://easyhealthoptions.com/who-are-cancer-quacks-now/
e. http://www.naturalnews.com/033847_chemotherapy_cancer_
treatments.html
224. Dr Mathe "stay awayfrom cancer clinics". concise,
interesting: http://cancertruth.org/Quotes-Mathe.htm

225. Dr EH Wilmer PhD: Very interesting. Includes AIDS:
http://www.whale.to/c/willner.html

226. Dr Leonard Coldwell. See his book, ref 29.

227. Chemo "therapy"extortion
a. Chemo is All About Money. Dr Glidden : (5m)

https://www.youtube.com/watch?v=k_Fzwj4Zpxs
b. Traditional Cancer Treatments cant work. Dr. Coldwell (8m)
https://www.youtube.com/watch?v=8xVYE9EZZ0g
Chemo, radiation cause cancer
c. **Video:** Every Doctor Knows Chemo Causes Cancer
http://tv.greenmednowinfo.com/every-doctor-knows-
chemotherapy-causes-cancer-says-surgeon/
d. http://tv.greenmedinfo.com/the-shocking-history-of-chemo-as-a-
cancer-drug/
e. Article http://www.drday.com/crs.htm
f. Dr Brawley, CNN Health Conditions expert.
http://thechart.blogs.cnn.com/2010/10/06/could-chemo-drugs-
cause-a-second-malignancy/
g. http://www.cureyourowncancer.org/chemo-kills.html
h. http://www.medicalnewstoday.com/articles/248661.php

Part III 2. THE WAR AGAINST CANCER

228. Dr Linus Paulins PhD, Nobel Laureate. War on cancer fraud:
a. http://www.pnc.com.au/~cafmr/online/research/cancer.html
b. Impressive biography: http://en.wikipedia.org/wiki/Linus_Pauling

229. Dr James Watson, Nobel Laureate, on National Cancer
a. http://www.blackherbals.com/no_more_pink_ribbons.htm
http://www.ssqq.com/stories/cancerfight01.htm
http://breakfornews.com/sickofdoctors/articles/medicalignorance.
htm
b. Background on Watson: http://en.m.wikipedia.org>title=James_
Watson

230. Dr Dean Burk PhD. Good article:
http://www.encognitive.com/node/1212

231. Carcinogenic breast scans:
a. "Screenings... with mammograms is unjustified...
it causes six (6) times more deaths than it prevents!"
Lancet (the world's most authoritative medical journal) 2000 355
pp129-134)
b. Screening mammograms do more harm than good:
http://www.canceractive.com/cancer-active-page-link.
aspx?n=1420
c. carcinogenic mammograms Sydney Ross, med. Anthropologist
http://www.breastnotes.com/bc/bc-causes-singer-mammoscam.
htm
d. report by Mr Mike Adams

http://health101.org/art_cancer_breast_myths.htm
USA govt health site:

e. http://www.ncbi.nlm.nih.gov/pubmed/1945480
f. http://www.ncbi.nlm.nih.gov/pubmed/374924
g. http://www.greenmedinfo.com/blog/how-x-ray-mammography-accelerating-epidemic-cancer
h. http://healthecancerblog.wordpress.com/2012/08/06/mammogram-madness/
i. https://www.med-ed.virginia.edu/courses/rad/radbiol/04stochastic/stoch-02-03.html
j. https://www.fredhutch.org/en/news/spotlight/imports/breast-imaging-in-symptomatic-younger-women--ultrasound-vs--mamm.html
k. http://campaignfortruth.com/Eclub/241105/CTM%20-%20paper%20on%20mammography.htm
l. good read. http://talesfromtheconspiratum.com/2013/11/25/shocking-study-spontaneous-remission-of-breast-cancer-found-to-be-common/
m. less mammograms=less cancer-Future Tech. Trends & their Likely Effects: http://www.futurepundit.com/archives/005744.html
n. http://articles.mercola.com/sites/articles/archive/2013/02/19/tomosynthesis-mammography.aspx
o. ***interesting "objective" article on cancer (breast, prostate etc) screening – Don't be misled by title and intro!!! You must read it ALL for a balanced view.
http://inspire2live.org/no-decision-about-me-without-me/
p. comparison of accuracy of 3 non manual & machine screening methods
http://www.drmostovoy.com/Thermography_Mammography%20.htm
q. New mammogram increases breast cancer: http://articles.mercola.com/sites/articles/archive/2013/02/19/tomosynthesis-mammography.aspx
r. Can You Cut Your Breast Cancer Risk by Skipping Mammograms?
http://articles.mercola.com/sites/articles/archive/2013/03/02/3d-tomosynthesis-more-risky.aspx
s. Dr Baylock. "Breast Cancer: Powerful Prevention Pointers every Woman Needs"
https://w3.newsmax.com/LP/Health/BWR/BWR-033-Breast-Cancer
t. Mammograms Can Increase Breast Cancer Risk:
http://www.dailymail.co.uk/health/article-392619/Mammograms-increase-breast-cancer-risk.html
u. http://www.greenmedinfo.com/blog/how-x-ray-mammography-accelerating-epidemic-cancer

232. MEMS, RFID
a. https://www.youtube.com/watch?v=PPsFXhyvGa8
b. https://www.youtube.com/watch?v=qCVVUuvXOoc
c. changes your dna-Christian-Forced implantation in Phillipinesvid (17m) https://www.youtube.com/watch?v=MxRuxtjal0c
d. Brave lady Soldier warning on RFID forced vaccination (10m): https://www.youtube.com/watch?v=aM8hpLlnz4o
e. Anonymous (3m) https://www.youtube.com/watch?v=aj2qaSJQqto
d. how to zap RFID (8m): https://www.youtube.com/watch?v=c0vZigwn09I
e. how to avoid: https://www.youtube.com/watch?v=V8PJpjkH780

Part III 3. THE HEART OF THE MATTER

233. Einstein quote on sacred gift and faithful servant:
http://www.goodreads.com/quotes/7090-the-intuitive-mind-is-a-sacred-gift-and-the-rational

234. a. https://archive.org/detils/solfeggioFrequencies-pureSineWaves-HelaingTones
235. 90% messaging is from heart to brain
a. www.myfoxdetroit.com/story/24239537/the-smart-heart-part-1-7-amazing-facts-about-the-hearts-control-of-the-brin

236. Not just electromagnetic wave. Heart more than just a pump
a. heartmath – http://tinyurl.com/oxvxg78
b. advanced reading – http://photonichuman.50megs.com/photo4.html

237 EM Machine
a. The eMwave2 machine: http://tinyurl.com/oxvxg78

238. Twin Slit Light Experiment
a. "Dr Quantum" animated (6m): https://www.youtube.com/watch?v=fwXQjRBLwsQ
b. Jim Al Klili (9m) https://www.youtube.com/watch?v=A9tKncAdlHQ
c. Quantum Theory and how we affect Reality (1.16m): https://www.youtube.com/watch?v=dD21gAkEOBw

239. Potential effect on world greater than a cell (a little you)
It takes one person with an idea to change the world; everybody else follows.

240. Human cancerous parasite (10m):
https://www.youtube.com/watch?v=C0R6EvtGnoE

241. Finally, Another Dr Emoto Masterpiece.
Messages from Water and the Universe.
"Essential" for coffee table and a perfect gift to a Best Friend!
http://tinyurl.com/lyy2kzn

Part IV
Additional Practical. Encouraging and Inspiring Resources.
To cut book size and cost to you, additional resources, mostly free, are available on http.//cancerfree.cf and the books that Heal newsletter.

Good Books
a. Change your Eating Habits! The How, Why and the (fun) Way! Recommended for those that want a change but lack the will, the discipline, or the knowhow! A highly successful worldwide program! http://tinyurl.com/pje3m6t
b. Dr.Schreiber,-MD,PhD.-Anti-Cancer, A New Way of Life
    http://tinyurl.com/k8psa6l
c. Timeless Secrets of Health and Rejuvenation.
    Andrea Moritz (Ayurvedic)   http://tinyurl.com/pbf6gcy

   Andrea Moritz (Ayurvedic)   http://tinyurl.com/pbf6gcy
   Videos a. Rupert Sheldrake and Bruce Lipton – A Quest Beyond the Limits of the Ordinary (1h.31m).
   https://www.youtube.com/watch?v=MQxcFL1uuk8

● At the time of going to press, the following eight (Holistic & Alternative) doctors have been found dead. Authorities point to murder and suicide! – Makes one think!

http://www.collective-evolution.com/2015/07/28/8-doctors-now-dead-holistic-alternative-authorities-point-to-murder-suicide-but-why/

Notes

Printed in Great Britain
by Amazon